MY PROSTATE DIARY

DOES IT STAY OR DOES IT GO

STUART ALEXANDER HAYWARD

CONTENTS

Copyright ©2023 Stuart Alexander Hayward all rights reserved. No part of this publication may be reproduced, distributed, or transmitted in any form or by any means, including photocopying, recording, or other electronic or mechanical methods, without the prior written permission of the author, except in the case of brief quotations embodied in critical reviews and certain other non-commercial uses permitted by copyright law.

Other than permissions granted, for privacy reasons, some names, locations and dates may have been changed.

Book Cover by Stuart Alexander Hayward

First Edition 2023

WARNING

Started writing today Tuesday 29th August 2023

Before going any further reading this book, I try to be honest and tell my story as it happens giving the details no matter what they are. There will be swearing and references to bodily parts and functions that may offend. If things like that may offend you then you're reading the wrong book. I will talk about upset and go into detail about how upsetting this was for not only myself but mainly for my family and friends. I wear my heart on my sleeve and it all goes in to this diary. This book/diary is mainly intended for men that have or are going through the process of finding out if they have prostate cancer, but it may also help anyone on their journey of finding out if they have the big C even if its not in their prostate. It is written sometimes from memory but mostly as a real time true story that I went through on my prostate cancer journey. I hope this will help people on their journey to understand the stages that I went through, to find out I had prostate cancer. I hope it will help and give people an inside on understanding how painful it is for family and friends to hear the news and may help anyone with cancer or waiting to find out if they have cancer to formulate their plan on how they break the news to their loved ones.

My biggest hope is that any man that is reading this wherever he may be that hasn't been to the doctors yet but thinks he should, gets the phone or just moves his arse and makes a fucking appointment at the doctors.

Just do it please.

GENTLEMEN IT IS SIMPLE ANY PAIN OR DISCOMFORT, IN OR NEAR YOUR KNACKERS GO TO THE DOCTORs. YOU ARE NOT BIG, STRONG OR CLEVER IF YOU DONT. IF YOU DO, IT MAY JUST SAVE YOUR LIFE.

INTRODUCTION

People used to say wait while you hit forty it's all downhill from there.

I was fine all through my forties. But my fifties fuck me that's a totally different story.

At fifty-four I was still going regularly to the gym and although not huge or massively strong I now look back and realise I was at a decent level of strength and fitness for my age and physical size.

Then I injured my right shoulder. The pain was a bit of a dull ache but steadily got worse until it impacted on nearly everything to do with lifting or even putting clothes on especially on my upper body.

The range of motion in that arm due to the shoulder injury became very limited and very painful in certain positions.

I paid for various treatments including sports massage therapy, Cryo therapy and I even bought a vibrating massager but all to no avail, until I eventually went to the doctors and found out I had torn a ligament in my shoulder.

I am still in the process of getting this sorted as I start this prostate diary just to give you an in-site on my general health.

Due to the shoulder, I virtually stopped going to the gym but did and still do go out on my bicycle mainly up to the allotment which is also good for a bit of general digging and pottering about for a bit of fitness. No biking in the winter or if it's raining in the summer. Soft lad yes, I am, same with golf, I only play if it's nice and dry, although saying that if im out and it does rain I will stay out doing whatever it is that I'm doing.

I work four days on four days off doing two twelve-hour day shifts followed by two twelve-hour night shifts with four days off (three and a half really as you get up about 12/1pm off the last night shift).

I also still play golf again as mentioned only in the summer months when it's nice, but I can tell how my fitness is not what it was, and those hilly courses take it out of me.

I have Duputrens disease in both hands which is the tightening of the tendons causing lumps in your palms and the restriction of movement in your fingers causing them to bend in towards your palm. I've not researched this to find out if it's hereditary but my father has it and my brother so who knows maybe it is.

I've had a cortisone injection in my shoulder about three months ago which did help but now it's nearly as bad as it ever was.

I made the decision to start getting more serious at the gym again as my fitness was and still is not where I would like it to be. I have lost a lot of muscle mass due to not going to the gym and gained a decent fuking rop to be fair. But at fifty-six am I that bad? I do see men of my age in a lot worse condition than myself but I also see men in better condition so I suppose I'm not doing too bad fitness wise but yes it could be better.

So why start a "Prostate diary" in the first place or at all?

Well, most people that know me know I write poems, verses and the odd ditty or song if you like. Now to start with a few years ago the writings used to get a bit of attention on Facebook, but it's calmed down a bit now, which is fine. Sometimes I may write something that people can relate to and that will get some feedback, but I think now the writings are more like little stories and people may or may not like them, but I enjoy writing them and post them anyway.

I have been asked why I write them and to be honest it's something I don't really understand. I could be sat at home, up at the allotment or even at work it doesn't matter where, once something clicks in my head it could be about a word a feeling an event or anything else really. Once it's in my head and I have the first few words or a sentence then I must write it down. If I don't start writing it down within the first few minutes of thinking about it, then I will forget it and normally it doesn't come back it's gone.

The funny thing is that when I start writing I can sometimes think about the initial subject or thought I've had but then the poem or verse can go down a totally different path and end up totally different to what I thought I was going to write about in the first place.

A strange thing I find as well is that after writing something I often read it and think where did that come from, have I just written that.

Anyway, I digress, and I will say now during this journey however long or short it may be there will probably be a lot of digressing along the way.

For anybody that is old enough to remember, I used to love watching the two Ronnie's with my dad. One of the best bits I remember was Ronnie Corbett used to sit in a big armchair by himself and tell a story. In this story he would go off at all tangents with stories in stories coming to a final funny ending, I used to love watching him tell those stories so maybe I have a bit of Ronnie Corbett instilled in me who knows. I am hoping for the happy ending at the end of this story, but we will have to wait and see about that.

THE BOLLOCKS

So that's the introduction finished, and I don't think there's been a mention of the prostate, yet which is the star of the show. Well, we're not there yet.

If anybody does ever get to read this then it is men that I hope will get the most out of it and if it saves someone's life, then that would be amazing. For all the women out there, this may give you an insight as to what's going on in a bloke's head that you may know or love that's going through the same experience. This may help, it may not, you will have to read it and find out.

This next paragraph or two are fresh from today. What you will read next is jumping forward in the story a couple of months but it's what happened today and it's only today I have started the diary. I have thought about doing a diary a few times over the last month or so and never got around to it, but I will tell you what actually made me start writing this in the next paragraph or so.

Today was my hospital appointment to have biopsies removed from my prostate. I'm an Electrician by trade and along the years in plying my trade there are certain qualities you gain and or learn. One of these is to not panic and to therefore keep a level head which then enables you to make the right decisions when under pressure especially if people around you are panicking. Where does this come in you may be thinking well, I'll tell you shall I? Today I was and still am shitting myself, but my wife thought it was because of the procedure. The procedure was a scary thought I must admit that, but reading up knowing what's going to happen to me allowed me to analyse the information and stay cool and calm letting the doctor do what he had to do without panicking beforehand and so not getting upset and ending up in an emotional state.

So, I said I was and still am shitting myself which means I am very scared not actually shitting in my pants. Scared of what then, I've had the biopsies done which I will explain about in more detail later but that wasn't scary to me. Some people are terrified of hospitals, and I must admit there not my favourite place. If you're in one and not visiting or escorting someone, then there's a good chance you've fuking hurt yourself or suffering some kind of illness or are having a procedure or operation done. None of these are fun but I would assume probably necessary.

The procedure didn't scare me but what could be in the results does cause me some concern.

Back to the hospital appointment later.

So, Bollocks is the title of this chapter, what exactly have bollocks got to do with the prostate in my case apart from the obvious biological reasons.

For a long time now, I have suffered on and off with pain in my testicles or what I believed to be pain in my testicles. Pain in my testicles is where this story starts.

A few months ago, I started to feel pain in my left bollock which would come and go but then the pain started to be there more often virtually every day. I mentioned it to my wife who knows about my history with this and therefore told me to get to the doctors. As most men are stupid and think they will be ok, I did what most men do and waited a week or three or four then finally went to see the doctor at the appointment my wife had made for me.

I've not been at this surgery very long but I have to say this doctor looks quite old, I'm not good at guessing people's ages so I won't bother but he has what I would call an old school attitude and he was and is a breath of fresh air in my opinion to doctors I have seen before.

GENTLEMEN IT IS SIMPLE ANY PAIN OR DISCOMFORT, IN OR NEAR YOUR KNACKERS GO TO THE DOCTORs. YOU ARE NOT BIG, STRONG OR CLEVER IF YOU DONT. IF YOU DO, IT MAY JUST SAVE YOUR LIFE.

Now on the build-up to making the appointment my father who has been treated for prostate cancer and bowl cancer which left him with a stoma and a bag had been getting on at me for quite a while about my age fifty-five then, fifty-six now telling me I should get the PSA test done for my prostate gland.

PSA, Prostate Specific Antigen test is a blood test that tests specifically for the prostate antigen as the title says. This value I believed went from one to five.

Today after speaking to the doctor, I now know it can go much higher and there's no real cap to it, it all depends on how healthy your prostate is to how high or low your test result comes back. Although less than three is deemed to be good it can be a false reading as a high score can mean nothing and a low score may hide the fact you could have cancer. So, the PSA test is sometimes frowned upon depending on which doctor you see.

So, my wife makes the appointment and I go see the doctor. The appointment is for pain in my left testicle which I thought was probably better than it being the right testicle as that is the bigger one and may have hurt more. The strange things we men think, because it was the small one, I actually thought if I have it removed at least I keep the big one which would be a result. Anyway, I'm at the doctors and he's looking at his computer screen as I walk into his surgery.

"Is it Mr Hayward" he says.

"Yes, doc good morning how are you" I reply.

"Sit down" he says pointing to a chair at the side of his desk, "you're having pain in your left testicle" he asked.

I sat down and mentioned the pain in my testicle, but I had also had pain in my abdomen which I had been a bit worried about so with my father pushing about the PSA test I thought I would mention that too.

After the initial pleasantries the Doc was straight into the business no messing about, old school you see.

"Stand up then" he says.

So, I stand up.

"Pull ya trousers and underwear down" he carries on.

I pull my jeans and pants down to my knees and stand there with my Crown Jewels just hung there, ready to be examined.

He started to feel my testicles and nearly straight away found the pain-full area on or very near the left bollock.

"Whoa that's it Doc yep your bang on the money yep steady doc bit tender that" I said in probably a voice a few octaves higher than normal.

"You have Epididymal cysts. We used to drain them in years gone by, but we don't do that anymore" he replied.

"Oh, ok so I just live with them then Doc" I asked.

"Yes, nothing to worry about" he said.

"While I'm here can I just mention, I have been getting abdominal pain as well doc and my dad has been getting on at me to get a PSA test done" I was saying and before I got chance to elaborate any further.

"So why didn't you say that in the first place instead of beating about the bush and wasting time", he says straight to the point.

"Uh well my testicles are painful, but I just thought I'd ask about the prostate test while I was here" I said rather sheepishly.

"Sit down put your arm on my desk" he says.

So, I put my left arm on his desk and within a minute or two he got out a tourniquet wrapped it around my upper arm stuck a needle in a vein in my arm and took a vial of blood. If you don't hear anything don't worry, it's fine otherwise the hospital or surgery will be in touch.

"Thanks doc much appreciated", I said and left the surgery thinking, well that went well fingers crossed and that is where the bollocks came into the story

AFTER THE BOLLOCKS

I'm shit at remembering dates, years and I'm especially shit at remembering names. I've worked at the same place now for over fifteen years and I call more people "mate" or "love" because I can't remember their names it's terrible and can be very embarrassing. After I'd had my first blood sample taken as I've just said I can't remember how long after, but it was only days I was contacted by the doctor's surgery and was told there was nothing to worry about, but they needed another blood sample.
I did ask why I had to have bloods taken again and the lady who I was talking to from the doctors said my reading may be a bit high which happens often for various reasons, so they wanted to take another.

When the doc took my first blood sample, he stuck the needle in just above the crease between my forearm and bicep. Sharp scratch and nothing to worry about the doctor did it with minimal pain and only left me with a tiny bruise you could hardly see. To be fair I don't bruise easily, if I get a bruise, I've had a decent knock. It was the day of the second blood sample, so I went to the docs. At this doctors they have a method of seeing the doctor which starts off with you getting a number. You get your number you then sit down and must ask the people in the waiting room who has the number before yours, so you know who to follow in when they come out after seeing the doctor.

This time I didn't get a number I was just told to sit and wait in the waiting room, and I would be called when it was my turn. About ten to fifteen minutes later a nurse came and called my name, so I followed her into her room and took a seat. I am not scared of needles but obviously given the choice I'd rather not have to encounter them. The nurse asked if I preferred an arm and I just replied, "no preference really which ever looks the best for you".

When the doctor stuck the needle in as I said previously, he went in with the needle just above my crease from forearm to bicep and it didn't really hurt or leave a bruise. Oh my god the nurse stuck the needle in right in the middle of the crease and it fuking hurt. She moved it while it was in my arm to get it in to the position where she could get the blood out of one of my veins which didn't seem right to me. She took the blood put the cotton ball on the hole the needle had made then held it in position with a piece of the stickiest tape that's ever been made and off I went. Later that day I removed the tape which pulled all the hairs out of my arm it was stuck to and nearly removed the skin as well. You may grin you may not, but it hurt more than the frigging needle. I can just see all the women reading this now thinking try waxing you soft lad.

The next day I woke up my arm was a little sore where the nurse had stuck the needle in, and I had a lovely bruise joining my forearm and bicep.

Again, if you don't hear anything all is well otherwise you will be contacted.

This is where my memory is shit again, I think it was the actual next day or two days after they rang me up and asked for me to go to leave a urine sample. By this time, I'm starting to get a bit of a worry on. Off I went to the doctors again, collected the vile/container whatever it's called went to the bog and filled it to the top without spilling a drop and missed all my fingers, result. Very happy with my self-handed it to the receptionist still warm.

The following week I get a phone call saying the pee sample is ok, but I must go and give another blood sample.

I'm now thinking is this good or bad I haven't got a clue now, am I on the borderline, or are they just trying to get a low reading then I don't have to have further treatment.

I made a date for the appointment and waited for it to come around.

The day came I went to the doctor's surgery, and I was called by a younger nurse than before. Now I'm thinking oh here we go I hope she knows what she's doing she only looks young. She was lovely, very polite, very professional and she didn't leave a bruise. Don't judge a book by its cover comes to mind. So within about five to six weeks I'd probably been to the doctors more in this period than I had previously through the rest of my adult life.

I started this journey at fifty-five years old and now I'm fifty-six. I work continental shifts and feel fuking tired all the time getting old is no joke, but I do believe it is a privilege because there are a lot of people who are not lucky enough to get to even my age let alone retirement age. Don't get me started on the retirement age and the fuking government that keep putting it up.

The following week, one day I got home from work, and I had missed two calls from the hospital on my personal mobile. Due to having a works mobile provided I leave my personal mobile at home. I had the phone number for the hospital reception from ringing about a torn ligament in my right shoulder. Yes, I am dropping to bits but that's another story for another day. It was nearly seven o'clock that night when I noticed the missed calls so I thought I would not bother trying that night I would call from work the next day.

After several calls of just being left on hold I managed to get through to the urology department who then told me I needed to contact the X-ray department as my bloods had been checked and it looked like I needed an MRI scan.

"MRI scan, fuking MRI scan what's she on about" is going through my mind when I realised, I'm still on the phone, "hello, hello are you there Mr Hayward" I heard the lady say.

"Sorry love, yes, yes I'm here" I replied rather shocked and a little disoriented to be honest.

"Have you got a pen and I can give you the direct number to call just in case no one answers and then I'll transfer you through" she added.

"Yes, I've got a pen" I replied and promptly wrote the number down as she said it to me down the phone.

I think I rang that number over ten times with no answer.

I eventually rang the hospital reception and asked if they could put me through to the X-ray or MRI department as I had been trying for over two hours with no answer. Unbelievably they picked up straight away. That might be one to remember in the future. A lady answered the phone, and she was very pleased to hear from me as she had tried to contact me to try to get me booked in, but I had not answered my phone. She booked me in for the following Tuesday at a time I can't remember. You would think I would remember things like that, but I told you my memory is shit. So, I'm booked in for an MRI scan and now things are getting serious and quite real. Thinking about it now, I realise why I was surprissed when I was told I needed the MRI. During the time I was having the bloods taken I had not really thought about what would happen if the blood tests gave a high reading. Subconsciously I must have been hoping I would be ok and therefore thinking bad things would not help so I didn't.

THE MRI SCAN

There's one thing I will say at this point an Electrician I used to work with had his prostate removed and my dad had his treated. My dad also has several friends that have prostate cancer, and some have had treatment and they have had it return. I will be honest here up to now I have not googled anything about prostate cancer or the treatment for it. We have phones, laptops, iPads and lots of other devices that can bring all sorts of information on a screen for us to analyse and scare ourselves to death with, if we want to. I have chosen not to go down that path and to listen to the doctors. Now I know there are horror stories of doctors getting things wrong and I get that, but my dealings so far with my local surgery doctor and the Barnsley hospital doctors and nurses I have to say have been exemplary in my opinion absolutely brilliant. So apart from what I have heard or been told by the people I have mentioned, that is all I know about the treatment of prostate cancer.

But what I did google for research purposes due to the fact I'm a sparky is info about the MRI(magnetic resonance imaging) scanner. This machine is awesome it is basically a big magnetic camera, but unlike an x-ray machine it does not use radiation and the images are taken in slices normally three to five millimetres thick in the area the doctors want to examine. I mentioned it is like a tube and fuck me it's not a very big tube to be honest.

On my MRI appointment after getting into one of the sexy gowns they provide, I went into a room and was asked to sit on a sort of bed in front of the MRI scanner. Whilst sat there because the area I was having scanned was specifically for my prostate I was informed that my bowls may move about and cause the image to be poor quality so I would have to have a cannula in my arm which had a drip fitted feeding a drug into me which stopped my bowels from moving enabling the scanner to get good images. Here we go again another fucking needle but to be fair I was used to them by now and needles didn't bother me anyway it's just some are inserted better than others. When you're walking around with a great big bruise in the crease of your arm looking like a smack head, it's not a good look. I think the nurse said the drug was Buscopan, again I haven't researched it that's just what needed to be done so crack on.

The needle was in my right arm, while the drug was flowing I was asked to lay down and given a little device to hold in my left hand which was on the end of what looked like a thin probably 3-4mm in diameter flexible cable. This was the panic button. I was told about how noisy the machine would be how it would take a while and would get very noisy. I was offered some headphones which I welcomed. I was asked if I felt ok and if I was ready to go into the machine. I was all good to go I put the earphones on adjusted them accordingly and gave the nurses the thumbs up.

The bed you lay on is motorised so as soon as the nurses left the room, I could hear what I assumed were motors starting to do their thing and I was slowly driven into the scanner.

When I was young my mates and I would get into all sorts of scrapes and situations. Some of them I think about now and I shake my head in disbelief. I'm now in my mid-fifties in a hospital totally safe laid on a motorised bed being driven into this tube scanner. It can't have been more than an inch and half maybe two inches maximum away from the tip of my nose. I didn't think I was claustrophobic, but this made me think about maybe I was just a little bit. This I did not like at all. The MRI machine was tight I had a tube from my arm with the cannula needle in it that started to pull on my arm making the needle hurt which I thought was going to get ripped out of my arm and the panic button which was also being pulled but I wasn't letting go of that. As I got about halfway in the tension on the needle stopped and on the panic button too. The slack must have just been caught and then must have freed off or something. It was at about three quarters of the way in my nose started to itch and at this point I really started to believe I may suffer from a fucking fear of tight spaces. "FUCK ME I DON'T LIKE THIS", I'm thinking. My heart was pounding louder than the music playing from the earphones. I needed to gain control, or I was going to panic.

"What the fuck are you panicking for you bell end get a grip you're in hospital it's not going to squash you", and then I realised where the panic was coming from.

Not sure if you have heard of the Titan submersible. But a few months ago, this tube-shaped submersible vehicle made of mainly carbon fibre went on a voyage down to the titanic. Yes, the titanic which is very deep. Anyway, there was a massive search as they lost communications with the sub and long story short it imploded killing all five people inside. It would have been instantaneous they would not have felt a thing apart from the terror before that point if they knew what was coming. So, this was the trigger that was making me feel so scared.

After giving myself a good talking to, apart from the itch which was annoying I calmed down and let the machine do its thing. I was in there quite a while if I were guessing I bet it was going on for half an hour but then it might have only been five minutes I don't really know. One thing for sure I was glad when they got me out of the bloody thing.

Once I was out, I sat up on the moving bed removed the headphones and the nurses removed the needle and asked if I was ok which I was.

I got talking to one of the nurses and asked her if they got people that panicked because that was tight and not very pleasant. I also mentioned the itchy nose which I gave a good scratch as soon as I was able to on removal from the scanner. She did say that yes indeed people did panic pressing the panic button to come out and one of the reasons a lot of people pressed the panic button was because they had an itch they needed to scratch.

All done and dusted so that was the MRI scan over with, just a matter of waiting for the results again.

I mentioned earlier that I write poems or verses whatever you want to call them and due to the MRI scan, next you'll find a poem that came from that experience. I did post this on Facebook but due to the fact I didn't want people to know about what's happening at this point I didn't put any references in about my prostate journey.

FEAR

There's nothing to fear but fear itself
But that's easier said than done
Fear comes from many things
Some you know there in your mind
Other fear comes that's not so kind

What is fear and how does it work
It's that feeling of dread that you just can't shed
Some may tremble shake or sweat
You can't control your feelings of dread
The blood runs fast it pumps in your head

Some feelings of fear maybe dreams there so clear
You wake up wide eyed
Grabbing your partner by your side
These are nightmares that you've had
Sometimes screaming like your mad

But what about the fear that freezes you stiff
It maybe your just standing looking over the cliff
When the fear triggers it's hard not to shake

But is the decision really yours to make
When all that you feel is your life is at stake

So do you grab the spider or pick up the snake
Because fear is real when you start to shake
So how do you conquer this feeling of dread
Keep away from the spiders that lurk in the shed
Somethings that scare you are worse in your head
So just look a bit deeper into what causes that dread

Stu

GROWING UP

As a child growing up let's just say we didn't have all that the kids have to play with today to get their fun so we went outside to play for our fun and some of the places we used to play shall we say we're not the safest. The MRI scan brought back a memory of me playing out in the street when the drains were being re-laid all the way up our street and on through the fields beyond.

Basically, the work men were digging a trench which was probably about eight to maybe twelve or so feet deep. In the trench they were laying concrete pipes that were about three feet internal diameter. Now back in the day the health and safety back then shall we say was not as keen as it is today. All they put around the trench was just a wooden fence held together with wire. It wasn't very strong or very rigid. Due to the fence being weak this meant we, my mates and I could take full advantage of this and just get to the trench and pipe work whenever we fancied using it as an adventure playground.

One day we were playing out and there was a stretch of pipe that had been laid about thirty metres long. We could get into the pipe at one end but couldn't get out at the other. I had saved some bangers from bonfire night, so my mate and I hatched a plan. There were I think five or six of us that went into the pipe. It was tight but not as tight as the MRI machine. We crawled in on our hands and knees and you could see the light at the end of the tunnel so to speak but it was still quite dark inside the concrete pipe.

My mate and I let the other lads get in first and we followed behind. While we were in, we started talking about what if the pipe collapsed, we would all die or be stuck and starve to death if we weren't rescued in time. We were about halfway through, and our mates were just about near the far end of the pipe. We sat down with our backs against the pipe wall our feet on the pipe in front of us, and we then got the bangers out. We lit one each and threw them in front of us screaming "the pipes blown up get out quick".

Fuck me I am not kidding the noise from the bangers was deafening we nearly shit ourselves and we knew what was happening. I thought for a moment the fuking pipes were going to crack, cave in and we were all going to die. The lads up front all turned around because the end they were at had a steel wire mesh against the end stopping them getting out. They started to move towards us on knees, hands and the ends of their shoes or whatever footwear they were wearing. I thought I was deaf and all I could hear was a ringing in my ears then I saw the lads coming towards us at full pelt. My mate started to try and tell them it was us that had set of some bangers, but they weren't listening and to be fair I'm grinning as I'm writing this. Their faces were pictures of pure terror and eyes as wide as saucers, we were putting our hands up shouting "it's ok stop, stop", trying to get them to stop but they weren't having any of it.

They were like spiders crawling at warp speed and ran straight over the top of us and didn't stop. I just started laughing and my mate did too we laughed until we had tears running down our cheeks. Back to the diary.

THE PROSTATE BIOPSIES

Last night I was on a night shift at work and spoke to my manager who I had told about my diagnosis from the MRI scan on my first day shift of this rota. He had agreed that I could go home at eleven o'clock that evening due to the fact I would be up at seven the next morning. My original biopsy appointment was at nine o'clock, but someone had cancelled so I was first in at eight o'clock sharp on Tuesday 29th August.
I was to turn up at the urology department ward thirty-eight floor eight. From there the procedure would be done in the X-ray department on the ground floor.

I think my wife was probably more worried than I was and was able to come with me as she was off work until she started her new job tomorrow.

We arrived bang on time if a few minutes early, so we stood outside the ward doors until they were opened, we were then allowed in. We were shown the way to the waiting room and we each took a seat, then we while I was called for.

A very nice bloke came who I assume to be a ward nurse.

He called my name and off we went to his office. We sat down and he asked me questions to ensure I was who I said I was, and he made sure that I knew what I was there for. He gave me two tablets which he explained were antibiotics just in case I got an infection from my back passage into my prostate. I swallowed the tablets, and he drew a very good diagram showing my kidneys, bladder, prostate gland and my back passage where the doctor would get access to my prostate gland. I have to say you are a star mate. What a lovely bloke doing a great job. He made me feel at ease while explaining the nitty gritty of the procedure.

When we were sat waiting for the nurse there were others in the waiting room area consisting of another couple with the bloke probably a similar age to me maybe a bit older. If your younger than me mate I apologise I am shit at guessing peoples ages. There were also another two blokes on their own who were collected before the nurse arrived just leaving my wife and I and the other couple.

We were sat close to each other, so it was hard not to hear what the other couple were talking about. His wife was talking about what was going to happen and I overheard him talk about the biopsies. We were sent some paperwork and after going through the procedure he like myself had read in the paperwork that the doctor would take upwards of twenty biopsies from our prostates. The bloke had his paperwork in his hands and didn't look like he wanted to let go of it any time soon. I'd left mine at home.

Both of us had returned to the waiting room after taking our tablets and talking to the nurse, then a nurse came called both our names and the four of us followed her to the lifts.

We exited the lift on the ground floor and followed the nurse to the X-ray department. Our partners were shown chairs in the waiting room, and we were to follow the nurse into the procedures waiting room. She gave us one of the stylish gowns each and told us to strip down to our socks and shoes and wear the gown. The changing rooms were at the side of the room she got the gowns from.

We got our gowns from the nurse picked a changing room and got changed. I had an elasticated arm, green gown that was like a surgeon's scrubs. I have a bad shoulder and can't put my right arm behind me, so I struggled to tie the gowns ribbon around me. I came out first then the other fellow followed not too long after. He looked a bit more nervous than I was so I tried to make lite of the situation and said, "I didn't think we would make it on the catwalk", to which he replied "I think my back ends all hanging out" which made us both laugh nervously.

"Do you need me to tie you up buddy I don't mind", I asked.

He looked uncomfortable and replied, "no I'm fine I'll manage".

We were sat across from each other and he didn't look like he was in the mood for talking. I was feeling ok to be honest but didn't continue to talk to him as he looked petrified and not in the mood for small talk, so I left him to his own thoughts and sat there quietly minding my own business.

"Mr Hayward, if you'd like to come this way Mr Hayward", the nurse said. It was the same nurse that had brought us down from urology earlier.

I got up looking rather splendid in my surgeons green elasticated armed scrubs and followed her into the procedure room, well I suppose thats what you would call it, I dont think it was an operating theatre. There was a large wide screen monitor on it with what I thought to be my MRI scan on it at the right side of the bed and all the gear to do the procedure on the left hand side of the bed.

Now this doctor, he is a top man as well, this guy is sticking things up people's arse holes probably every day he's at work, it's his job. He's a professional arse hole prober. He asked me to sit on the side of the bed and explained what he was going to do. He also told me why I was having the biopsies done. He told me that one of the his colleagues had examined my scan results from the MRI and had decided I scored a four. This score this time did only go to five and he said he had checked the MRI scan and scored me at 3-4 which still required biopsies which is why I was here. Top man, spoke to me like I was his best mate brilliant, lovely bloke. He made me feel at ease as much as someone could, that you knew who was going to stick something in where only things should come out, but that's just me.

"So, Mr Hayward, I am going to take some biopsies from your prostate today. I will be taking about six to maybe eight at the most", he started saying to me.

Before he carried on,"ohh right doc I read it was upwards of twenty or more that would be taken in the paperwork I was sent, so I'm happy with that", I butted in with, and with that he had a slight chuckle and told me it wouldn't be that many.

"I will ask you to lay on your left-hand side in the foetal position with your backside on the edge of the bed. I will use a lubricant and insert a probe and apply an anaesthetic first into your prostate to numb it. You will feel a slight discomfort before it goes numb and then I will take six to eight biopsies. When I take the biopsies, you will feel a pushing and then hear a bit of a noise. I will let you know before I take each one. I have your MRI scan on the monitor over there and I will have a live view on my screen from the ultrasound probe here behind you. I am aiming for an area of about eight millimetres in diameter and I will take about three or four samples from there and one or two from each side of that area. The procedure won't take long. You have had antibiotics already due to the area we're taking the biopsies from. If you feel hot, sweaty and dizzy like you're getting a cold or feel flu like symptoms due to an infection after the procedure it will happen within the first day or two. If this happens you must go directly to the Accident and Emergency department and tell them what procedure you have had done. They will put you on an intravenous drip, with antibiotics in it to fight the infection. You may get blood in your urine, your faeces and your semen. Normally your urine and faeces will clear in a couple of days, but your semen could take a week or so" he explained very clearly, I thought.

"Are you ok to go ahead with this", he asked me.

"All good doc, do what you have to do buddy no problem", I

answered.

"If you would just lay on your left side for me then with your backside just over the edge of the bed", he asked.

I laid on my side and stuck my arse out over the edge like he asked. I'm thinking fuck me, not literally but I didn't get a look at the probe he's going to stick through my rusty sheriff's badge, so I have no idea what the fuck to expect. So, I'm thinking if I stick my arse over the edge and get my knees as far up to my chin it might make it easier for him to get it in and less painful for me.

That morning when I got up, I had a nice warm bath before setting off. I made sure I gave my bum hole area a good clean with the nicest smelling shower gel we had. Well, I wanted to be nice and clean for the doctor. I did consider trying to clean inside my bum hole but didn't consider that for long. My wife wanted me to shave all my arse cheeks and into my arse crack, but I told her to do one. Hairs growing back on your knacker's itch enough, I wasn't shaving my arse, and I didn't think it was that hairy that it would cause the doctor trouble getting the probe through it, it's not like it was a forest of arse hair.

"Ok I'm going to apply some lubricant and you'll feel a pushing sensation as I insert the probe", he warned me.

I think I actually said, "cheers doc", what the fuck was I thinking.

Anyway, he was right I felt the lube, cold and wet then a bit of a push and he was in.

Somehow, we got talking about the extension he was having built. About how all the prices had shot up it was ridiculous. I told him about one of the lads at work who was also having an extension built and he said the same since before Covid to now his quote was over fifteen grand more. Tiles don't even start on the price of tiles he had told me. I had also told the doc I was a sparky and that I worked for a large bakery in the area that made exceedingly good cakes. I went on about the robotic machinery we have and the many different lines of automation and products that we made on them. He had asked me why I hadn't brought him any cakes which I thought under the circumstances that would have been a good idea to keep him onside or sweet you may say, but anyway I hadn't.

During our quite detailed talk of building prices, he did take some biopsies.

"You're going to feel me push a little and then a little noise and that will be the first biopsy", he said to warn me again to be ready.

To be fair it was more the thought of what he was doing than what he was doing that was the worse bit. It didn't really hurt but yes it was slightly uncomfortable. My wife says she thinks things like that are degrading. I disagree, the doctor is doing his job and for me he did it very well and there wasn't a point through the whole procedure where I was scared or didn't know what he was going to do to me next. I think he took six or seven biopsies, and he was done in probably ten or so minutes if that. When he took the biopsies, I could feel him push like he said and then it was like a crunch type sound but that was it really, nothing really painful just a bit uncomfortable, it sounded a bit like a stapler when he took the biopsy.

"That's it Mr Hayward we have what we need", he said.

"Nice one doc did you hit the bull's eye", I asked him.

"Haha yes, yes, I did. I'll just clean up and I'll show you", he replied.

So, when he inserted the probe into my little brown star it didn't feel like he had gone that far in, but when he was removing it, it felt like he was pulling the garden hose pipe out of my back passage.

He removed the probe wiped my bum for me and asked me to turn over and lay flat on my back for a while as I may feel a bit dizzy or sick. I turned and laid on my back but felt fine. I had a few minutes then just said I was ok could I get up, he said I could, so I did.

"You asked if I'd hit the bull's eye", he said to me smiling.

"I can show you if you would like me to", he asked.

"Oh yes please doc that would be great", I replied instantly.

He pointed over to the screen situated on the right-hand side of the bed and we walked over to it.

"This is your MRI scan, I can move the image forwards or backwards and each one of these images is a slice of your body. Let's have a look at it yes it says there look three millimetres. The images can be three millimetres or five millimetres yours are three. If you look there, that's your bladder and as I move this way your back passage and now your prostate comes into view. That's the middle of your prostate and the outside there is shaped like a horseshoe. If you look at your right side, it's clear and quite a white area but if you look at the left side of the horseshoe it's dark and not as clear. That's where I've taken the samples from and a few from around the edges", he explained.

Wow, I love technology, pcs, machinery and tech devices always have and im luckily it comes with my job. It was great him taking the time to show me as he didn't have to, and I thought he went above and beyond. He had explained that the area he had taken the biopsies from could be a myriad of different infections, it didn't always turn out to be the big C.

I asked him about the position of the area he needed to get to, and I was a little lucky in the fact that my target area was at the bottom of the prostate near my anal passage. If it had been at the top portion of my prostate, it would have meant a bit more pushing and maybe a bit more discomfort to get to the area to take the biopsies.

I did think it was good of him to show me but sometimes maybe too much information can be a bad thing. I'm no doctor but that left side didn't look very fuking good to me. But I suppose like I say I'm no doctor and we will wait for the results hopefully it's a couple of weeks on tablets and the infection goes away, happy days. We will see.

On my way out of the procedure room the other fellow was sat there in the same chair with the same worried look on his face.

"If you don't want me to say anything mate then just say so. I will just tell you it wasn't as bad as I thought. Honestly don't be worried he's a great doc and he was great with me mate try not to worry be over in no time", I told him.

He just looked at me with a wry smile and then just carried on staring in front of him. When I looked at him, I did wonder if he was thinking whether the doctor had cleaned the probe properly after it had been up my shit box because that would have gone through my mind. With that I went to the water drinks machine and poured myself a drink of water. The doctor had told me to drink water and I must have a pee before I was allowed to go. If there was a large loss of blood to report it to the nurse or if I struggled to have a pee, I may have to go back up to the urology department. I wondered what they would do up in the urology department if I couldn't pee. I started to think if I couldn't push a pee out would they push a pipe up my pipe so to speak and so I started gulping the water down. About five minutes or so later I went to the toilet a little apprehensive and pushed out a wee. No real pain and no blood I could see with my bad eyes. Flushed the bog washed my hands and went to find my wife.

Terry my wife was sat in the same seat she was in where I'd left her earlier before my procedure. She was sat talking to the other guy's wife or partner. I came along from the corridor saw them and smiled. They both saw me at the same time, and they looked like they had been having a real heart to heart conversation. My wife seemed ok but the other guy's Mrs looked teary eyed and very upset. Terry gave her a hug and we all said goodbye and hoped that our journeys down this road would be healthy ones and cancer free.

Turns out the women had been having a right old natter. The other guy had basically gone through a similar journey as me to end up here in the hospital. His wife had told mine that his PSA scores were both over eight and so he was sent for an MRI. His wife also told my wife that his MRI score was a clear four. My fingers are crossed for you good buddy hope we are both going to be fine. So that was it the biopsies done. Now it's just a waiting game again for what will be the most important test results of my fifty six years on this planet so far.

WEDNESDAY 30TH AUGUST

It's the day after my biopsies we're taken and last night was my last night shift of that four on. The shift was busy, and I was in a little discomfort but nothing to be really bothered about. My first few visits to the toilet for having a pee didn't show any signs of blood that I could see but then my peepers are not the best in the world and there was no pain maybe a little ache. No signs in my poo as well which was a bonus although the first time going for a number two was a little scary to be honest.

Throughout my night shift it did feel like I was leaking from my back passage, and it felt like I needed to wipe my arse all the time. On visiting the toilet, I would find that my bum hole was clean and all good which again was a result.

My wife went for a health check today before she starts her new job tomorrow. After this she got home just as I awoke from sleeping after my last night shift. She fancied a walk, so we put the dog in her doggy push chair and off we went. She got the doggy push chair as our dog is 14 years old on lots of medication and struggles to walk. After saying all that just like the young ones say these days the dog is living her best life as we are spoiling her rotten.

Down the dirt track past the big school and along the canal banking was our route then down the pavement along the side of the main road to the top of my parents' street and on we went to my parents' house. It was cloudy with intermittent bursts of sun shining through every now and then, so it was quite nice for a walk.

We put the dog still in her doggy push chair in front of their house front door, rang the bell and hid around the side of the house. My mum opened the door to see our Misty just sat wondering where we had run off to.

"Ohhh bless hello love what are you doing in your pram you come for a walk love" was the greeting our Misty got from my mum.

We then came from around the corner and was greeted just as warmly.

We ended up in their back garden where my dad can normally be found pottering about on some project, he's started to keep himself busy in his shed. The shed has more lean than the tower of pizza and I believe he may have built it before I was born.

We stayed for a while and you're probably thinking what the hells he blabbing on about. Well I only had the biopsies taken yesterday and the only people that know about my current situation is my wife, my manager at work and one other work colleague who I work with every day and would say he's a good and close friend who I can trust to not tell anyone and who I can confide in as he can with me. So, we are talking in my mum and dads back garden when my dad started telling us about some more appointments, he had been informed about today by a hospital letter regarding his stoma. My parents are both now in their eighties and news of me having problems with my prostate is not news I think they need carry. So, I questioned my dad about his experience with his prostate. To be honest I did feel a bit guilty not telling them about my issues and then talking about my dad's prostate cancer and quizzing him for info.

My dad when he was about sixty-six maybe sixty-seven was going to the doctors then the hospital to have his gall bladder out. On returning to the hospital someone had put in his notes to check his prostate scores from his bloods and from this they had found his prostate had a cancerous tumour.

So, he turns up to the hospital to see the doctor about his gallbladder when the doc says "sit down Mr Hayward, I'm sorry to tell you that you have prostate cancer".

This hits him like a thunderbolt. Shortly after he found out he let people know telling my brother and myself first before everyone else. My father worked all his life very rarely having a sick day and is someone I think very highly of and whom I love every hair of his balding head. When he came to tell us, I was in my thirties so still quite young compared to now in my mid-fifties. Even back then my dad was someone who I looked up to and I don't think I had ever seen him scared or really upset about anything.

When he told us about this cancer, I could see he was terrified. We all tried to comfort him and told him it had been caught early and he would be ok. Luckily, he was and since then he's had fuking bowl cancer during bastard Covid and had to have the eight-hour operation with no one allowed to visit him before or after the operation while in hospital. Never complained once just got on with it, proper hard core.

Told you I could go off on tangents but the bit that sticks out that I get from my dad's story is that he was actually lucky that he had the gall bladder problems because this probably saved his life from prostate cancer. Also, the fact it was found early gave him options for his treatment type and great odds for full recovery of which he had.

His choice of treatment was the radioactive balls that are injected directly into the prostate making him radioactive for twelve months while directly killing off the cancer. Great bloke my dad top man.

We ended up going in a pub in Royston which is where my mum and dad live. They still live in the same house they lived in when I was born which is probably going on sixty years now.

We had a few pints and a bag of crisps or two then set of home which is about a mile or so away from the pub. The weather was still nice, and the dog was still living her best life bless her.

Did the usual when we got home which was have a bath, ate tea, watched telly and went to bed early to watch more Netflix in bed while we got sleepy.

While we're in bed I was feeling ok and fancied some sexy time. Big mistake.

After we had made love, yes made love because I am an old romantic. After sex if you like that better, my wife turned the light on to go the bathroom which is downstairs in our house and then I saw the blood. My wife also saw the blood and I saw the look on her face. She looked scared and had a little go at me saying we should have waited, asked was I ok, and did it hurt but I said I was ok, and she left it at that. There was quite a lot of blood in my semen which did shock me a little to be fair. I had been warned about it but because I hadn't had any blood in my pee or poo, I thought I was good to go. I was wrong, the blood was there and there was quite a bit of it. What I didn't expect was the pain afterwards. I had pain for an hour or two until I fell asleep, and it carried on into the next day, basically from waking up, it was there but a few tablets took the edge off. I told my wife I was ok but in all honesty it did hurt quite a lot and was very uncomfortable.

SUNDAY 3RD SEPTEMBER 2023

Back to work today after my four days off. Since we had made love the day after the biopsies, I had been suffering with a bit of pain in my abdomen in the prostate area. I assume it maybe the making love that caused some of it, but I do think there was probably going to be some sort of pain afterwards from having something like that done anyway, so sex or no sex I thought it would probably hurt anyway. I keep telling my wife I think we're good to go again now for sexy time and she just looks and shakes her head at me. What's that all about she won't let me near her the miserable cow. Hope she doesn't read this because if she does, I've got the furry side coming my way, I'm only kidding she doesn't beat me, she locks me in the cellar. No, she doesn't I'm only kidding it's a joke.

Last night we had a curry and there were a few chillies in what I had. Even though I have the same dish most of the time from the same place we use for our Indian takeaways different chefs put their own little twist to the recipe and this was hot.

Last night I had a bit of tummy ache and didn't sleep well after the takeaway. Today at work I had a lot of pain in the same area I'd been getting it in since the procedure and couldn't make up my mind if it was bad guts or prostate pain. About an hour into the shift a visit to the loo answered the question although there was still a bit of ache there.

So apart from a bit of aching every day it's been ok really, it's just waiting for the results that's the hard bit now. So, I'll be back to carry on the story when I get the results unless anything interesting happens before then that's worth putting in here.

MONDAY 4TH SEPTEMBER 2023

It's been nearly a week now since I had the procedure, and I am wondering if my prostate is still bleeding. The doc did say it could be a week or so before it doesn't show in my semen. My wife has been very supportive through all this but me losing blood like that I think did shock her. She has been asking how I am every day and to be honest I'm fine. The procedure was uncomfortable at worst, I think we do more worrying and make things seem worse than they are especially when your health has anything to do with the C word.

I have still got blood in my semen but hopefully that's the last of it.

Maybe we will hear something this week.

THURSDAY 7TH SEPTEMBER 2023

Last night was my last night shift of this rota and it was a hot sweaty long, horrible bastard of a shift. My work mate the other shift Electrician has been off all four, so it's been a long four shifts. I had tried to get to talk to my manager about still passing blood but could never get him on his own. My workmate the other sparky had messaged me asking if I had heard anything which I still haven't, I let him know there was no news yet and thanked him for his concern. There in that moment was my justification for not telling anybody that doesn't need to know, until they need to know if at all.
I had been plodding along getting on with normal everyday life as you can't really do anything else. I hadn't really been consciously thinking about the results I suppose it's easier to not think about them for me. Some people would be in a state worrying and fretting everyday but that's not me.

If my wife ever worries or frets about anything I always say to her if you can't change what you're worrying about there's no point worrying, what will be will be. Handle the situation if or when it happens. I know that's sometimes easier said than done and we are all made differently after all.

Back to my mate's concern.

I had read his messages and replied after waking up in the afternoon after my first night shift and never thought much more about it other than I mentioned it to my wife, and she agreed it was thoughtful and showed his concern for my welfare.

I got to work and started to realise I was feeling a bit down.

I had been writing one of my verses/poems the night before on my work phone whilst on my break. It was all but finished they normally only take me five minutes to write. We had done our hand over and I had put my work phone on charge. Anyway, I let it charge for a while then put it in my pocket. A little later we were talking about a machine, and I had answered a breakdown call on my phone so while I had it in my hand, I thought I'll read my poem out aloud. There were only two work mates present and one was not in conversation, so I read it out to the other. This guy obviously doesn't know, and he has commented previously about my poems being negative. I read it out and I will write it after this for you to read and make your own minds up about the negativity but obviously you will know the journey, I'm on he doesn't at this point. He looks at me after I read it out shows me his wrist on one arm and with the other hand makes it look like he's slitting his wrist that he's held out towards me.

I just looked at him and thought what a fuking horrible thing to do. Yes, he doesn't know what I'm going through but why do people have to be so thoughtless and nasty without taking other people's thoughts into consideration.

I got up and walked off keeping well out of his way for the rest of the shift.

Through the rest of the shift, it was apparent that my sparky work mates' message had hit home on what I was going through and what I could have up and coming from a telephone message or a letter through the letter box. Up until last night I hadn't had a wobble, this was the first and the confirmation for me that the less people that know the better.

In fact, thinking about it if I had gone public with the news from the beginning I could be getting messages like that on a daily basis you would never be able to get it out of your mind explaining to people what's happening and telling them if you had or hadn't had any news. That doesn't sound fun, and I can hear people saying you selfish prick, friends and family deserve to know. Well, it's happening to me and I'm dealing with it my way and when I'm ready to tell people if there's anything to tell I will.

I suppose there is already quite a lot to tell really, so all the people that are or will be interested will find out soon enough.

Here's the poem and it still doesn't mention the star of the show. I'm sure I will write something poem wise with prostate in it sometime soon. I normally post most things I write on FB but this one is just for you. Please don't slash your wrists after reading it it's only a poem.

TIME

Nobody knows how long they have

Will you reach 60 years

Will you reach 80 years

You don't know when you will go

You may be young you may be old

Live everyday like your last I've been told

For if you're lucky you will grow old

You try your best to keep yourself fit

You're out on your bike your lifting weights in the gym

You've also considered starting to swim

Is this too much though don't you think

With your fat belly you're not going to sink

Strava on your phone counting the miles going by

Smartwatch on your wrist counting heart
beats adding more data to your list

Peddling hard sweat pouring out

Look where you are you know you've gone too far

How you wish you had the car

Sore again from the gym you only went on a whim

Buttocks sore from the bike might be softer on a trike

Don't stop now you're doing so well

Just keep putting yourself through hell

The miles you've done you could go to the moon

Even though your Sixty soon

So if I keep on riding my bike

Pumping the weights and fishing for pike

Will I live until I'm 90 is that old can I still karaoke

Just keep doing what you do

Eat the food and have a poo

Drink the wine just make sure you make the toilet in time

Live your life the best for you

How long you have is not your choice

Doesn't matter how loud your voice

Your time will come be certain of that

You don't have nine lives like a cat

Enjoy this one it's as simple as that

Stu

FRIDAY 8TH SEPTEMBER

Not heard anything yet it's Friday and my wife is on a six o'clock start. Both my wife and I had a bad night's sleep with the weather being so warm. I was awake at four o'clock my wife had been up 3 or 4 times for a pee waking me up every time she went to the bog. I woke up at four could not get back to sleep so surf the internet on my ipad until my wife gets up at five ish and went downstairs. I set my alarm for 10.15 for whatever reason and eventually get back to sleep. My alarm goes off and I snooze once or twice then get up and out of bed.

Today is the leaving do of our Engineering manager, so I've got plenty to do. I have some breakfast and walk to the gym. The gyms about a mile away in the next village and it's very warm so it's a sweaty walk. Smash the gym to bits for a fifty-six-year-old and walk back home.

Got home sorted out the clothes I was going to wear later and ran the bath.

Time was passing me bye and I hadn't washed the dishes from the previous night's tea. Washed the dishes checked the bath which had nearly flooded over so I turned off the taps pulled the plug to let some water out and stripped off my clothes. After my bath I put on my clothes I had ironed before getting in so got dressed and was ready to go. It has been absolutely red hot all week after 15 minutes I was sweating like a pig on a spit. My shirt was ringing wet, so I went upstairs to my wardrobe and changed my shirt.

One of the lads was picking me up at quarter to two and it was half past one, so I was in front time wise, with plenty to spare.

He rang asking if I was ready which I was, and he promptly picked me up.

Off we went headed to the town centre for our managers leaving do. We get into town parked up and said goodbye to his son who was taking the car home and meeting us later. We set off to meet the lads in the Brahmers boozer in town and all was good.

We had been walking for less than a couple of minutes and my phone started to ring. I have an I phone, and I had my I watch on. I get shit loads of nuisance calls but because I'm waiting for a call from the hospital, I've been answering them all instead of cancelling the calls. So, we're in the town I haven't got my glasses and I feel the call on my I watch vibrate. So, I accept the call on my I watch and put my watch to my ear. I tell my workmate I must take the call and hang back letting him carry on towards our destination.

"Hello, is that Mr Hayward" the lady asked.

"Hello yes, it is", I replied.

I couldn't see it was the hospital calling until she said she was from the Urology department it could have been anybody.

I confirmed my identity, and she gave me a couple of options to attend the urology department for an appointment to see the doctor.

I'm out in the town walking to the first boozer and I get the dreaded call. My work mates in front of me by thirty feet and I've just taken what's probably the scariest most important phone call of my life so far.

"Come on bell end who you talking to we're out out", he calls.

"Coming Jesus, it's not my fault I'm wanted", I replied.

We carried on to the first pub and my head was spinning.

The lady on the phone never said anything about the results of the biopsies and I never asked. So really it could be good news, or it could be bad. Now I'm writing this at home slightly pissed having been out on a great afternoon/night leaving do.

So, we get to the first pub and my head is spinning a little thinking are you fuking joking me, it's Friday afternoon could you not have rung me Monday. But would I rather have had that call today or Monday and the answer is today without a doubt. So, we're in the first boozer and people are arriving every other few minutes to have a few beers and wish the main man all the best. Now I've made the decision not to make my circumstances public and I stand by that but today with all those people I know from work not having any idea of the phone call I've just taken I have to say it was not easy. We had had a few beers, and I was thinking if I just get everyone's attention and just shout out, I might have the big C it would all be out there and no more keeping it secret. Then I thought again and that would not have been a good idea so obviously I made the right decision keeping quiet.

The guy who's leaving do it was, is a well-liked bloke and he will be missed. I've worked in this job for fifteen years, and I have been to many leaving dos. This one I think is the first time I've ever seen a factory manager turn up. I have to say even before buying everyone who'd turned up a drink, he is a very good and well-liked factory manager and from the time I've dealt with him he seems like a decent bloke. I had downed a few pints and messaged my wife about the hospital appointment but without my glasses I couldn't see her reply, so I went off to the toilet upstairs and rang her. As I was talking to her the factory manager came walking bye and gave me the wink and put out his fist to say hi and I replied with my fist to his and a hi with a nod and a wink back to him.

Any earlier and he may have seen me with tears in my eyes and several little salty water droplets running down each cheek.

Back to the group I went and enjoyed the drinks and excellent company.

I'm on my days off now and Monday is my first day back on shift. Monday morning is my appointment with urology, so I need to let someone know preferably my manager but we're out getting pissed.

There's a big group of us out and getting my manager on his own to confide in wasn't going to be easy. I'm stood talking to one of the lads when my manager comes along stands at the side of me grins and asks how I'm doing. I don't think he was expecting my answer. I nodded my head for him to lean over and he leant his head towards mine so I could talk to him without anyone hearing our conversation. He looked and I think he knew what was coming before I said a word. I told him I had just been called by the hospital and my appointment was for Monday morning so I wouldn't be coming to work did I need to call someone Monday morning.

"No, you've told me message me, so I remember cos I'm going to be pissed just do what you need to do I'll sort it. Don't worry about work just let me know what you're going to do not a problem", he said to me instantly.

We then had a conversation about my circumstances and that he'd been talking to his wife who like mine is a worrier and the fact that she had been getting on at him about if I was ok or not and that he should be ringing me.

We have a lot in common and do confide in each other especially with family stories. I have a great deal of respect for him and know I can tell him anything and it stays there with him as he knows he can with me. We obviously tell our wives that goes without saying. I had spoken to my wife and that was a great help and I know she would back me up through thick and thin but it's also nice to talk to one of the lads and get a "ahh you'll be rait mate what's up don't worry you'll be fine", to settle the nerves.

We all must work to pay the bills unless you're lucky and have retired the earlier the better. The fact that my manager said don't worry I'll sort it just let me know what you're doing was a big relief and takes away stress about work you don't need in these kinds of circumstances.

I think it was about nine o'clock not too sure to be honest, but I'd drank enough felt drunk enough and had had enough. The hospital phone call I think had probably played its part, so I rang my wife, and she was on her way to pick me up. A few people had already left, and some make a bigger exit than others. Don't get me wrong I can milk a goodbye as good as anyone but not tonight. So, I just tried to slip of around the back with no fuss and got caught out.

"Oi Hayward where are you going", was shouted at me with a few more besides all with varying words of obscenity.

Oh, bollocks I'm thinking I just want to get off. Anyway, the few lads that saw me including my manager were a bit pissed off that I was leaving but he gave me the wink and said, "good luck let me know what happens", which was nice to hear and meant a lot.

I set off outside and saw my wife in the car so jumped in and we set off home.

My wife and I got home, and I went through the evening's events. We obviously spoke about the phone call and again I struggled with it to be honest.

The lady who rang didn't give any information away as to what the appointment was for. It's obviously for my biopsy results but I have no idea if it's good news or bad. Would it be better if she had said your results are back Mr Hayward it is cancer can you come to the urology department next week. That's not the call you want but when she doesn't say your results are back and your all clear then it's going through your head it's the first one, but I suppose on Monday morning I'm going to find out either way.

Anyway, it's three minutes away from midnight I'm sobering up and my head is banging like a broken gate in a storm. So, I will say good night and the next instalment will probably be Monday afternoon, you will hear from me then goodnight.

SATURDAY 9TH SEPTEMBER 2023

Back earlier than I expected, and I will tell you why. Slightly hungover when I got up this morning at about half past ten. Ligged in bed for a while until I thought "well you have got to get up I can't stay in bed all day", when in fact if I had wanted to, I fuking could have, I'm an adult and I could have made the decision and just stayed there. But I didn't, I got up had breakfast and went out on my push iron(bicycle). The last few days have been really, and I mean really warm and muggy. The sun was full in the sky and very little if no cloud. Was this a good idea, maybe, maybe not but I was going anyway. The plants at the allotment needed watering and I couldn't be arsed with the gym so the bike it was. Messaged my mate but he had put a shelf up in his garage after moving house recently so that was him knackered for two weeks.

So, what's this bike ride got to do with today's diary insert. Well on the ride I went a way that enabled me to go past an old work mates house who is retired now. Before he retired, he was diagnosed with yes you guessed it prostate cancer. The way I went meant I had to go up a decent hill of which at the top there's a nasty junction. Being on my bike I had cycled on the pavement as much as I could. The week before I had gone the same way and there were several blokes digging into the bank at the side of the pavement.

I was later to find out from my friend a guy had been killed after being hit head on by a van whilst riding home a quad bike he had just purchased. I managed to get up the hill and the sweat was leaking everywhere from me by the time I got to my friend's house which was across the other side of the busy road. His car and his wife's car were both parked outside their house, so I knocked on the door, also used his little metal knocker and within seconds he came from around the side of his house from his back garden.

"Now then how's things, what do I owe this honour to", he asked me.

"Well, I thought I better bob in and see how the retired people live", I answered. I laid down my bike behind his wife's car and we went around his house to his back garden and sat at his table where he had been reading a local paper.

I asked if he could keep a secret which I knew he could before I asked, and he'd replied that he could looking a bit worried. I told him my circumstances and asked him if he had any advice, and could he tell me his story if he didn't mind. I'm not putting his name in here people who know me and know him will know who he is.

His story is basically the same. He had the tests done, MRI scan then the biopsies. After the biopsies he was contacted as I have been to attend an appointment to discuss his results. He attended his appointment and was told he had indeed got prostate cancer. The advice he gave me was very good. He's been through it and came through the other side, but they found his early, so he was lucky if you call getting cancer lucky, but you know what I mean.

Things might have changed now it was five years ago since he had his diagnosis, but he said there were several doctors at his appointment and he was told about or offered several different treatments for his type of cancer, but it was his decision on which way or what treatment he chose. Although they had caught it before it had spread, he had a nasty cancer and he needed treatment immediately. He chose to get his prostate gland out and get rid. He went into hospital one day came out the next all done. He had exercises to do after the operation while in recovery but has been ok since.

While I was there, he had other visitors arrive, so we didn't really get to finish our conversation before I left but it was so nice to talk to someone who has been where I am and come through the other side. We had a laugh about the tests especially the biopsies and he had had the physical prostate check which I hadn't had so we had a bit of a laugh, and I thanked him for his time and advice before setting back off on my bike journey to the allotment.

Off I wen,t watered the plants up at the plot and then obviously had a lot going through my mind about our talk earlier so ended up just walking about and apart from watering some plants I didn't really do much more.

I'm sat in my back garden as I'm writing this today with a beer thinking things through. What's there to think about? Well, I'm getting a lot more pain now it's not more painful, but it seems to be more regular. This could be from the biopsies, or it could be that it's getting worse whatever it be either cancer or infection. At this point and after speaking to my old work mate who is a mate not just an old work mate, I do believe it will be a cancer diagnosis. I hope I'm wrong but if I am right then I hope we've caught the bastard early.

The one thing that has settled me after having the biopsies was that the doctor had said "whatever it was either cancer or an infection it didn't look like it was anywhere else", which got a big sigh of relief from me. My mates PSA test was only 2.6 and mine was 3.5 and 3.6 although the PSA test is not a definite test it's a good indicator.

I was wondering today after speaking to my mate about it all, how the other guy had gone on who was having his biopsies after me. His PSA test was 8 so he must have been worried. Our paths may cross in the future who knows I wish him well and all the best on his future and the journey he will take.

FUCK UP

uck bastard fuck bastard fuck, I've just deleted the whole diary and it's only up to here I've been able to restore it back to. It's now Tuesday the 12th of September so I've lost the last four days of writing, and I am fuking devastated. This is one of the best things I think I've ever done in my life. It could help so many people in the same circumstances as me and I've fuking lost the most important four days up to now in the dairy. I cannot explain how totally gutted I am. I will try to re-write the last three days and if you're reading this then I was happy with how it turned out. There has been so much raw emotion I just don't know If I will be able to get it anywhere near what it was, but I will try. As I have previously stated what I write goes down once or it's forgotten so let's see what I can remember out of the blur that I've just lived through. I suppose it just adds to the story. I'm writing this all on my iPad and I was trying to edit something and somehow selected everything tried to go back wiped the lot, panicked instead of pressing the reload go back icon I pressed the leave the file icon saving fuck all. I've gone to history and although it says ten minutes ago it's three days short. To say I've just had a meltdown would be an understatement. So, the next three days are going to be from memory and not that day's raw feelings as I lived them.

RESULTS DAY

Monday 11th September 2023

After two long weeks of waiting, it's here the day of the results. I'm in bed writing this and my wife is downstairs having breakfast. I don't want to get up I'm thinking that it would be a good idea to just stay in bed all day. Yeh fuck it I'm an adult and if I want, I can stay in bed all day, not do results day, not go to work today just stay in bed and have a do fuck all day. Grow up, get up and get a grip you bell end we find out today if you're going to see Christmas this year. Get your arse out of bed and fuking move it. So, I did. Got up, got dressed went downstairs had a bit of breakfast and was ready to go. Appointment is at 9.40am it's 8.45am "come on Herbert it's time to go", I said to my wife. Herbert is a nickname I call my wife, some of my mates and especially my brother as it was him, I believe who originally set it off in the first place, I think.

"It's too early we'll be there way too early if we set off now", she replied.

"Will we bollocks it's going to be busy at this time, there's traffic lights for road work's everywhere and then we will have to wait and queue to get a parking space in the hospital car park", I said back to her. After I had said that we promptly set off.

As I had predicted, we hit road work traffic lights and had to queue at the entrance to the hospital car park to get in. The hospital car park is a one out one in system when full, but it let us in, and nobody had left so we had to wait for someone to come to their car and leave the car park to give us a space to park our car in. We had our ticket, parked up and set off to the lifts in the hospital that would take us to ward thirty-eight on the eighth floor, the urology investigations unit.

We got to the eighth floor and followed the appropriate signs until we were sat in the waiting room bang on time I might add. I hate being late for anything. I would rather be twenty minutes early than two minutes late, that's just how I am and how I've always been to be fair.

We had not been there long when a nurse came and called my name and asked if we would follow her. She took us around the corner into a corridor where there were two chairs waiting, so we sat on them at the same time that she pointed at them, and it looked like the doctor's office was the door just off to the right of us

"Thank you", I told her.

"You're welcome and the doctor will see you shortly", she replied with a nice big smile.

We weren't doing much talking now my wife and I but, in my head, I was thinking about all sorts of shit that the doctor could possibly tell us.

The same nurse came back a few minutes later and asked us to follow her into the doctor's office introducing herself again and the doctor and his name of which I could not tell you either of their names. I know, I know my memory is shit I keep telling, you must believe me by now.

"Please sit-down Mr Hayward and you, is it Mrs Hayward, how are you today", he said as he greeted us and shook my hand.

"Thank you. Well doc, I'm ok but, I could be a lot worse or a lot better in ten minutes depending on what you tell me next", I replied.

"Ok, its good and bad. You do have cancer in your prostate gland, but it's a very low risk cancer and doesn't need treatment at this time", he said.

He then went on to tell us that from my biopsies there was only one that had got cancer cells in it. From this they had deduced with my MRI scan than it was low risk, it hadn't spread, and I would not need treatment at this moment in time. I would be monitored with regular blood tests for PSA with a telephone call discussing the results and any further action if required. If these tests were ok and not showing any further increase in cancer activity then after twelve months, I would have another MRI scan to see what the cancer was like and decide where to go from there. If there was none or very little change the three-monthly bloods would be extended to a length of time decided by the MRI scan results. He then went into possible treatments and why they prefere not to treat the cancers if they are not causing too much pain and are obviously not life threatening as the treatments are so damaging to your body they would rather not.

My father in-law had cancer and was treated for it. He died due to the amount of cell damage that never stopped after the radio therapy and chemo that he had to get rid of the horrible disease.

He was going on about a catheter in my penis and it just wasn't registering.

"Uhh sorry doc what was that I uhh just missed that bit it's gone over my head", what had happened was that I had gone 'cancer deaf'. This is what I now call what happens to you when you're being told about cancer. When someone drops you the C word, it makes you go cancer deaf, and you hear nothing but blah di blah di blah. Cancer deaf I think it may catch on.

So, the doctor repeats himself for me and my wife also tells me in the other ear what he had said because she was still listening bless her. I did get it the second time around, well a little bit in between "blah di blah C….A…..N….. cancer then, that's what he's on about to me", I was thinking.

He then prescribed me some tablets which I was to trial and

see how they reacted with me. He said these were to loosen the muscles around my prostate area to help me urinate easier giving me a better quality of life. They would reduce the amount of semen I ejaculate as some of the semen would go up into my bladder. Who the fuck thinks of these tablets and then works out the recipe to make them, unbelievable. Not sure if I've mentioned this but I don't like taking tabs so that could be a battle, although my wife may think differently. Oh, and they may lower my blood pressure and make me feel ill. If that happens, I can stop taking them, if my fuking heart doesn't stop first. Best thing is I don't have a problem passing urine just a little push to start with then I'm good. Anyway, we will see what happens with them I haven't picked them up yet.

To be fair what a result we all knew there was something there, the scan and the blood tests had shown it the only better result was that it could have been an infection instead of the C word. So, we talked some more, he gave us some literature to read and made sure I understood what he had said. Which I had gotten the gist of it to be honest even through the cancer deafness.

Cancer, I have cancer a fuking horrible word that is a horrible disease. Fuck me I have cancer. This morning I was Stu, now I'm Stu that bloke with cancer, "is it prostate cancer he's got", they will say, fuking brilliant. My wife was proper hard core, I'm thinking am I missing something here how the fuck are you not ruined. We thanked both the doctor and the nurse, we took the paperwork, the prescription and went on our way to find the hospital chemist.

"You alright love", she asked me.

"Uhh yes I think so after what I've just been told", was my reply.

Not sure what I was or am still feeling. Initially it is shock you build yourself up for bad news like this but hope you never hear it. When you do hear it it's like you're outside looking in thinking do they mean me.

We found the pharmacy and handed our prescription over to the lady behind the counter.

"Do you pay for your prescription love", she asked me.

"Yes, I do, I'm afraid some of us have to", was my reply.

It always takes ages for the prescriptions to be processed at the hospital said the wife, so we went for a drink in the café at the bottom of the near bye escalator. We had been there for a while when I said I would go and check if the prescription was ready. The wife said it wouldn't be, but I went anyway. I got up from my seat and started to walk back over to the escalator when I saw someone I haven't seen in years. I'm not going to say his name, but he was a warm bugger back in the day thirty plus years ago. I stood there just staring at him and he was staring back but he didn't do or say anything, so I began to walk closer to see if I was right. Was it who I thought it was. I walked over and we shook hands and said hello. I sat in the chair by his side, and we had a catch-up chat. I bet you can't guess what he was fuking waiting for. Well bugger me you did that's right he was waiting to go to get one of his weekly doses of chemotherapy for bastard bone cancer. We chatted for a while I told him about my very recent diagnosis, and we shook hands and I departed. Well, my old mate I really wish you the best and hope you get through it because it sounded like hell. He was just sat there but he was a hard little bastard back in the day so I would think he would be giving the big C a real good scrap, good luck pal. It's true what some people say that there's always someone worse off than you. I've been diagnosed with a mild prostate cancer and twenty minutes later I'm talking to an old friend who's fighting bone cancer, wow, I think it's called perspective.

The tabs weren't ready, Herbert had to get ready for work, so we set off home and I would pick them up Wednesday when I came back for my shoulder appointment.

Well, I said the star of the show would turn up somewhere and here it is.

PROSTATE GLAND

I need to write a poem about my prostate gland

How will I do it I don't know where I stand

But the prostate is the star of the show

Have I to tell you why

I've been off to the hospital

And they had a little spy

My prostate is not healthy

It gives me lots of pain

Is it really poorly or am I just insane

I get my test results tomorrow

Will I be full of glee

Or teary eyed with sorrow

We will have to wait and see

I've had lots of needles they stuck them in both arms

They've taken lots of blood the tests they worked a charm

The numbers they came back with were not very pleasing

When they fuking told me I almost started wheezing

So, what is going to happen I really just don't know

But one thing is for certain it may just have to go

If I'm lucky with fingers crossed it's nothing really nasty

If the doctor says to me I'm sorry but it's past it

Then my prostate I say to you

Goodbye you're going in the waste basket

So it's not all bad it's glass half full fantastic

My prostate is poorly they have no doubt

It has the dreaded cancer

I just want to scream and shout

But it's the best that it could be

So don't you feel sorry especially not for me

No treatment needed

No removal

That comes with the doctor's approval

So raise a glass hip hip hooray

I am so thankful for today

Listen now to what I say

Please go and have a PSA

Stu

MY MUM AND DAD

We made our way to the car park and went to pay the parking ticket. We had the change between us and tried putting it in the machine, but the slot was jammed or something. Every time we pressed the reject button it dialled through to the security guard. He thought we were taking the piss. We told him we weren't pressing the ringer button to speak to him, but he didn't believe us. In the end we used a debit card to pay which was much easier and eventually drove off. On our way out we noticed the barrier was up, so we need not have paid anyway, but I do believe it goes in the hospital kitty which is fine by me. In the car we didn't talk much my head was just, well to be honest it was just numb, empty and full all at the same time. I wasn't really thinking any clear thoughts that I could say had any semblance of eligiblity it was just mush. I didn't know whether to be happy, sad, laugh or cry really. We pulled up outside my mum and dads and boy I hadn't fuking figured on how bad this was actually going to be.

The not telling people to protect them was it right or was it wrong? Should I have told them to lessen the impact, no, I believe I should not have told them, and I stand by that decision. Months of worry compared to an upsetting conversation had to be right for me and my family in my opinion. We went into my mum and dads house and my mum was in the kitchen, so she saw us come through the front door. We went through the hellos and welcomes then sat on the sofa in their living room. My dad came down from upstairs and sat in his single chair and mum sat in hers. We just started talking about the usual things, the weathers still warm the news is all shit on the tv just the usual things. My wife had been squeezing my hand as a go on then tell them for a few minutes, but I was just sat thinking how the fuck do you drop the C word into a conversation knowing that these two people are going to be destroyed when I do. So was keeping the last three to four months to yourself the best idea now. Yes, yes it was because instead of that several months of constant worry and stress it was going to be just one sharp shock. It was going to be nasty, I know but in half an hour we would all be in a place of understanding that I'm ok for now and it's a good result as cancer results go.

I had formulated a plan, and I was about to put it into place. I had been thinking about how I was going to break the news depending on what severity of cancer I was going to have to tell them I had and it went like this.

"Right then so I just want to tell you some stuff I am fine, it's all good I'm ok and nothing's going to happen to me", is what I started with. This got their attention straight away and all eyes are now on me. "So, I've had some tests and I'm ok really, I'm ok. We've been to the hospital today and I've got a mild version of prostate cancer", and fucking boom I dropped the C bomb.

I was sat across from my dad and saw his face just drain and his bottom jaw would have hit the fucking floor if it would have been long enough. My mum, oh dear my mum did not take it at all well, but did I think she fuking would idiot I am. I've just told them something that goes against how life should progress. Nature should be, adults have children, they all grow older together. If parents are lucky, they become grandparents and maybe great grandparents etc. Then nature takes its course, and the elders pass away for whatever reason eg. Cancer some other health problems whatever but that's how it should be. No parent should have to bare the loss of a child.

"Oh my god no son no god please no, not you as well not you oh my god no", and she absolutely sobbed her heart out. I had to drop to my knees in front of her to stop her from falling off the chair she was sat on. I wrapped my arms around her, and she was shaking like she had hyperthermia.

"Mam I'm ok, I'm ok listen to me I'm ok". I kept my arms around her, and she slowly started to calm down. When she had got to a steady sob and nearly stopped shaking. I pulled away and faced her holding her fore arms to steady her and kissed her forehead. I think if she would have been stood up on her feet, I think she would have gone down like she had been shot by a sniper's bullet. She was coming around a bit, but it wasn't going in what I was telling her she had gone "cancer deaf".

I think the only time in my life that I could possibly relate to this kind of emotional pain and stress was what happened after the birth of my first-born child my daughter Kara.

Kara was born on a Thursday at 14.56pm and I was overjoyed. The feeling you have when having a child is mind blowing. Kara came into our lives on a Thursday and my wife and daughter stayed in the hospital overnight, so I went back into hospital on the Friday to visit my wife and newly born daughter. Terrys friends from work were coming to meet our daughter and catch up with their friend, so I arranged to go in after they had been there a while. I was going in to see both of my beautiful girls then I was going to go into town to wet my daughters head and maybe end up a little drunk with beer and high on life. I turned up and her friends Angie and Shaz were still there playing pass the parcel with our daughter. My god she was and still is beautiful. I couldn't harm a hair on my children's heads and I'm not going to go talk about the sick bastards that do harm kids, but I can tell you this if it was anything to do with me they would suffer.

Anyway, I get to the hospital, say high to all the girls and I was going to try prize away my daughter from one of the girls when my wife looked at me and nodded for me to come to her side on the bed. So, I walked over, and it was like being cancer deaf.

"She's got to go for tests there's something wrong with her", she said.

I looked at her and thought is she on about our baby girl or one of her mates from work.

"Stuart did you hear what I said she's got to go for some tests, she's not pooing out of her bum it's coming through her mouth and nose", the wife went on grabbing hold of me trying to get me to listen and understand what she was trying to tell me. I'm still staring at her just thinking what the fuck is she going on about you poo through your bum not your mouth and nose.

"What do you mean love I don't understand you, how can that happen you poo from your bum", I still wasn't registering what she was telling me.

"A nurse is coming for her in a bit to take her for some tests", she replied, still holding on to me.

I tried to analyse the information she had told me and still talk to her friends who I also worked with, so I knew them very well. The friends left and a nurse came with an incubator on wheels. She was very young the nurse and didn't really look like she had a clue what was happening apart from she was picking up a baby. She may have well been from the Royal Mail. I will explain. We put Kara in the incubator and set off to the high dependency unit on the top floor. I was still trying to understand how you poo through your mouth when I noticed Kara was beginning to show little beads of sweat on her head and face.

"Is she wrapped up too warm she's sweating", I said to Terry.

Then before Terry answered I understood exactly what she meant because it was happening smack bang in front of me. This greeny black gooey shit came dribbling out through her mouth and nose. I fuking froze looked at my wife we both looked at the young nurse who just looked lost and useless. To be fair to the young nurse she shouldn't have been sent to pick Kara up in my opinion it should have been someone with more experience and a nurse that could have explained more about what was going on as we knew nothing, and neither did the nurse.

I thought my beautiful daughter was going to choke and die.

I looked at the young nurse "well do something she's going to choke" I said in a raised voice probably shouting at her. By the time we all stood panicking trying to decide what to do, Kara had basically pooed out of her mouth and nose, and it had cleared, and she was breathing ok. I also noticed that the sweat had nearly all gone from her face and head. I could go on with this story in a lot more detail, but I won't say much more I'm just trying to explain the fear, shock and dread a parent can feel through the pain their children may have to go through. My daughter had to have fifteen centimetres removed from her bowel from having an operation a few days old. She was laid in an incubator with pipes and wires coming out of her from everywhere with a bandage covering the cut across her belly where the surgeon went in to do his work, and we couldn't even hold her. These were the worst two weeks of my life up to now and I'm fifty-six. This pain is a hard one to manage but manage it you do and you must.

I am a person that would rather take the pain for others than cause pain especially where my family is concerned. I will and would take the pain, so they don't have to and that's why I didn't want to tell them until I had to, it's my way of protecting the people I love from being hurt and feeling pain that I can stop. Back to my mum and dad.

Mum had eventually calmed down to where she was able to listen to me and my dad was sat up staring at me with tear filled eyes. I don't think I have ever seen my father cry. He got very emotional when my brother and I took him to see his beloved football team Glasgow Rangers in his hometown of Glasgow for his 80th birthday as a surprise but again that's another story for another day.

I was now in a position where both my parents could and were listening to me and taking in what I was saying. I explained I didn't need treatment, why I didn't need treatment yet, the plan that the doctor had come up with for me going forward which was the blood tests every three months with action taken as or when required if any. We were there a while and then it was time to go, Terry had to get home to get ready for work. We said our goodbyes and left for home.

Our son had been messing about in his bedroom or got up late and was going to be late for a shift at one of the Witherspoon pubs in town so I said I would take him while Terry got ready for work. I wasn't going to tell my son Corey until later when he got home from work it wouldn't be nice telling him about my news before, he had to go to work so it would wait while he got back home.

While I was dropping Corey off Terry had rung her Mum who I do love dearly she is a lovely woman who I always call Mother instead of her actual name which is Christine. Terry had also rung her brother and her dad's girlfriend Lynn to tell them my diagnosis. My wife never told me how they took the news and I suppose I'm better of not knowing I have enough upset telling my side of the family.

Just going off on one again.

Terry lost her father to what everyone believes was the big C but that's not exactly what happened. Yes, he got cancer and if he hadn't, he would probably still be with us today, but he didn't die of cancer. Terry's dad Dave had throat cancer. He didn't die from that, he eventually died from the damage that continued to happen years after he had had the treatment. He had radio therapy which is a hard aggressive treatment along with chemotherapy as well. It was horrific watching him go through that. Dave, I loved you mate you were a great father-in-law and a great friend, miss you lots Dave we had some great family times together.

I got home still a bit blurry of what the day had brought so far. Terry told me who she had rung and who she had told the news to and then she left for work. I had to now plan in which order I was going to ruin people's days. It was about two in the afternoon, I think. So, I messaged my brother to bob in after work if he could. This could be a hard one because he would want to know why. I could have told him I had some veg for him from our allotment, but he could have said he would pick it up tomorrow, so I didn't I just said nip in after work. As I thought after I texted him, he replied "a up bruv we're in one car so Bern will be with me wats up n b bout 4ish", that's his exact text.

With "no worries lad nowt just nip in", being my reply. He answered again saying ok it would be about four when they would arrive.

I have to say we all do it now, the text messages we write and send to each other are bastardising the English language so much I'm sure we're all going to start and forget how to write proper words. Then there's the emojis and there a language to themselves. I bet you could just use emojis to have a conversation with someone. The worlds gone mad.

Bern is my brother's girlfriend, and Bern stand for Bernadette. They moved house a year or two ago and now live together.

I still had a bit of time before then so I would go to my mates he's just moved into the same village as me and was only a five-minute walk away. I hadn't been to his house yet so I would kill two birds with one stone.

Didn't take me long to walk to his house. I knocked on his front door and he answered and let me in. His house was built onto an old farm out house development and it is very nice. It's a funny shape but it's nice. We spoke for a minute or so and then I told him my news. His reaction was a good one.

"Your joking", he says with a look of shock and surprise on his face. "Yeh it's a fucking cracker of a joke isn't it. Am I fuck joking you muppet why would I joke about that", was my reply.

"For fucks sake, what's going on its fucking stupid", he answered.

Again, after the initial shock he took it quite well and the conversation soon got back to his problems and how the NHS was shit and he couldn't get anything done, but that's just him. He did offer any help he could give which I know if I asked there's not a lot, he wouldn't do for me and that works both ways.

That went quite well to be fair, when someone can talk about their problems over yours it did make it easier.

MY BROTHER

I was beginning to wonder whether my tactics of telling people I'm ok before I tell them I'm not, was actually working. The fuking cancer deafness wasn't making it easy for me at all. My brother and his girlfriend would be here shortly so I wasn't going to change my tactics now I would stick with it.

"Ey up bro, Bernie come in sit down. How's things", was my greeting to them as they came in through the porch into my living room. Don't be thinking I'm living in a great big ponderosa with five bedrooms and a swimming pool because of the PORCH. I live in a three-bedroom terrace house with a upvc porch we had built on the front of the house to have somewhere to leave our dirty shoes instead of the living room. The front door enters directly into my living room.

"We're good lad what's happening bro, you got us some veg", he asked.

"Ey up Stu you alright", Bernie asked.

"All good Bernie love thanks", I told her.

"Right, so I'm all good I'm ok right. I'm fine there's not a problem I'm ok. I've been for some tests n shit, and it's come out I've got mild prostate cancer", I said to them and waited for the cancer deafness to do its thing. There was a slight pause from both of them and my brothers face was, well, I could say a picture, but it wasn't the fuking Mona Lisa. His jaw dropped, Bernie looked totally lost and didn't really know what to say I suppose. Maybe it wasn't fair to put Bernie in that position, but I couldn't see a way of getting my brother on his own and I will apologise to Bernie when I see her, I am sorry Bern it wasn't nice for you to go through that.

"Uhh what, fuck me bro what's happening then how bad is it what's doctors say", he was in a bit of shock I think and it's not often if ever my brother struggles for words. So, we sat and talked and to be fair to both of them the cancer deafness struggled to do its work here. My brother and Bern had poked two fingers at the cancer deafness fuck you and fuck off, nice one. They asked all the prevalent questions and were actually able to listen and take it all in. I stressed again and again to my brother about getting his PSA done and it's especially important he does now as our father and his elder brother have both been diagnosed with prostate cancer. GENTLEMEN IT IS SIMPLE ANY PAIN OR DISCOMFORT, IN OR NEAR YOUR KNACKERS GO TO THE DOCTORs. YOU ARE NOT BIG, STRONG OR CLEVER IF YOU DONT. IF YOU DO, IT MAY JUST SAVE YOUR LIFE.

As we were talking my son came in returning from his shift at Wetherspoons in the town centre. We pretended to talk about something else and he went upstairs to his dump of a bedroom as I knew he would. My son would be next on the list to catch my c bomb fuck me what a day and the worst was yet to come for me on the telling people my news front, my daughter was not going to be easy at all.

My brother and Bernie came to a point where I think they were ok with what I had told them and were ready to go. They both gave me a cuddle said I would be ok and left. I was begging to feel drained, and I could feel my emotions building every time I went through the process of telling people about the cancer. What I was realising is that no matter what I said before I told them, until they asked me if I would be alright the cancer deafness would not let go its grip. Maybe I didn't need to spend as much time before dropping the c bomb explaining I was ok just drop the c bomb let them ask all the questions and job done. No, that was too much of a shock in my opinion.

MY SON COREY

Corey is my youngest child born July 2005 now 18 years young. He is now turning into a big unit, and I wish I could get him into the gym he would be a monster but it's just not his thing. He plays computer games, a lot but I won't say he's a nerd I don't think that fits, but he spends hour after hour day after day on that bloody computer and he is interested in very little else. I cannot really complain as he only takes after me as I was the same when he was born, and he's only copied what he saw. When he was small before he could read properly, he would amaze me on his games. It was probably an early Xbox he got first, and he would navigate through the game menus from memory faster than I could read the instructions on the screen. Corey has always been a thoughtful child and thinks things through. If he was ever naughty which was nearly never if you said you will get a smacked bum as a threat to him, he would just look at you as if to say so what do your best dad. But if I was to say to him that's it, I'm not your friend you've hurt my feelings then that would really bother him, and he would then respond to my requests to behave. Corey if he puts his brain into gear can be very thoughtful, but other than that you must ask him to do what you expect or want him to do. To be fair if I ask him to do anything I never get a no or any back chat he just does it with no fuss. I was hoping he would follow me into Engineering, but he's not interested. From being a young child, he has had Lego every single Christmas of his life and it didn't take long before he was building the kits without needing

my assistance, which as a dad didn't come easy and I have to say it did sting a little. The last kick in the balls I had from him growing up and not needing his dads help was only a couple of weeks ago. Two years ago, he wanted a games pc for Xmas, so I specked him one up with a bit of input from an old mate who is an IT manager and bought him the bits for Christmas. He could build it with my help if he needed it. I ended up going way over budget, but he never asks for anything and he had had a shit time through Covid, so he deserved to be spoilt. This pc is now nearly three years old and in the world of pcs three years old is ancient. I found out since his friends have upgraded several components in their units. My wife says to me one day, watch for a parcel coming it's Coreys graphics card. "Excuse me sorry what? He's ordered a graphics card without asking for my advice", I asked.
"Yes, it should be here today or tomorrow", she replied with a smile knowing exactly what I meant.

But then that's not the worst part of it, the worst part is that he fitted the bloody thing as well without my help, I am gutted. Just throw me on the scrap heap with a label on my back reading 'dad no longer needed'.

Ok then "Corey can you come downstairs please", I shouted from the bottom of the stairs.

"Why what's up", I got as a reply.

"Come down please I want you", was my answer to him.

He came down sat on the other sofa and I began my story again.

It's hard to gauge what Corey is thinking he's not very animated apart from when he's cursing online at his friends over some online game there playing.

I told him about the cancer, and he just seemed to take it in no real emotion which is normal for him to be fair. He did ask if I was going to be ok and that was about it. I said "ok son are you ok? Anything else you want to ask me? I am going to be fine", I told him.

"No, as long as you're going to be ok that's the main thing", then he got up and returned to his bedroom. I hope I didn't spoil one of his games. He may think about it for a few days and come back to me once he's analysed it in his own way. He is only eighteen, so it probably doesn't register highly on his things to worry about scale. I don't know, as I said he doesn't give a lot away, but he does care.

MY DAUGHTER KARA

This was the one person I was not looking forward to telling due to several reasons. The main reason being that I knew she would be devastated, and she lives sixty miles away so it would have to be done over the phone which meant I would not be able wrap my arms around her to calm her down and comfort her until she was ok because she was going to react like my mum. It would be an instant reaction and the cancer deafness would be here in all its glory basking in its evil bastardness.
I was sat on the sofa with my phone in my hand, it said Kara on the screen, but I couldn't press it. We couldn't leave her not knowing and wait until we got through to Hull to see her and tell her, the risk of her finding out was just too great. I had to make the phone call it was all I could and would have to do.

Ring, ring, "hello dad, you ok", she asked. It was just something she said when answering the phone, she didn't mean are you ok and I think she sensed that I wasn't, fuck me I was dreading this I was going to cause her pain that I couldn't take away from her. It's my job to take as much pain as I can for my kids, so they don't have to suffer any.

Just to fill you in on my daughter. She is what you call the A star student. Wall of fame at big school getting the highest marks in the school. A's in her A levels she is just a work machine. When she went to do her A levels, she was wanting to be a teacher. I was happy with that it's not what I would want her to do in this day and age, but I could see her being very good at it and going up the ladder to head mistress of a school no doubt in my mind. Yes, I would say that I'm her dad. Anyway, she changed her mind and wanted to be a social worker. No, no, no are you out of your mind was my reaction but I couldn't put her off. Three years later

she's got a 1st level degree with honours and is now working for hull council as a social worker. That's why she is sixty or whatever miles away.

She has just moved into a terrace house with a friend from university who she shared accommodation with through the three years at uni. I asked the wife if she had her friend's number to text her and ask her if she would be at home with Kara later. She replied yes, she would, and Terry told her she would be getting some bad news from her dad and would need her friend there for support. She said OK and would make sure she was there.

"I'm good Angel how are you? Busy day at work", I struggled and was feeling the long day now starting to take its toll. I think I was on the edge of just breaking down at this point, but I wasn't aware of it yet. We spoke about her day at work, and I had to just tell her there was no point going on and on I needed to tell her.

"Right sweetheart I'm ok I'm not going anywhere but I've had some tests ok but I'm fine I promise but I've got prostate cancer", and it was instant. Within milliseconds "what you've got cancer dad no really", she said, and she was sobbing her eyes out in no time at all. I was struggling with this now, but I had to hold strong do not crumble do not cry on the phone you will make her worse.

"Listen, listen to me Angel I'm ok, I'm ok, listen to what dads telling you I'm going to be ok really I am honestly I'm going to be ok", fucking hell this was worse than getting the results.

"But you've got cancer, I don't believe you dad", and she was heartbroken. Writing this I have tears running down my cheeks what a horrible bastard life changing disease. I don't know if there is any other disease or condition that has this impact. I suppose there are, and families and individuals out there will have proof of that I would imagine, but cancer is up there and if it's not top dog then it's fuking close.

"Kara, Kara calm down darling, calm down please. Dads ok I am honestly let me tell you what's happening. Just listen to dad calm down stop crying you must listen to dad", but I don't think anything was going to make a difference I just needed her to calm down and know I wasn't going to die, at least not for a fucking long time, I hoped.

She was sobbing and trying to ask me questions but not sure what to ask.

"Right ok, now you've calmed down listen to me. I'm ok we found it very early so it's fine. I don't even need treatment. Doctors are going to monitor me. I will have blood tests every three month and that's it. No treatment honest no treatment how good is that", I hoped I was getting through.

We talked for quite a while until she had maybe not fully calmed down, but she was in a state where I could leave her. She needed to talk to her mum now and go through it with her where she wouldn't hear my voice. Terry was working and was waiting for me to message her that I had told Kara, so that's what I did.

The wife rang me back later after talking to Kara. Apparently, we must have been talking too loudly the last time she was at home, and she had overheard something about us talking about the doctors, so she knew something was going on. She didn't believe what I had told her and thought we were hiding something from her. I messaged her later and promised her that we weren't hiding anything I had told her the truth.

RESULTS DAY NIGHT

What a day that had been. I was physically and mentally knackered. All the hard work had been done. A few close friends, some stragglers and work mate's tomorrow to tell and then I can start to accept the news myself and move on. It was only six or more hours since I found out and it seemed like a week already. I was drained, and I just collapsed on the sofa looking at the ceiling with a blank mind. I wasn't numb, I was, I suppose, a little bit lost. I suppose most people that get that first cancer diagnosis feel lost probably as angry as fuck as well but I was lucky my cancer was not a bad one and I hadn't been told it was terminal because how the fuck you tell people that, I cannot begin to imagine.

I was just relaxing trying to just not think about anything and chill for a while on the sofa when the messages started to arrive. There were only a few messages but that was the tipping point for me to just have a total release of emotion and a real meltdown.

The first message was from my brother in-law, and he is a great guy and I love the guy to bits. He was only a teenager when I started going out with his sister, so I've seen him grow from boy to man and he's a great man.

His text was a "sorry to hear about your news bro" text and that was like a hammer blow to my temple. People only send sorry messages when things are bad or bad things have happened. As I'm trying to control my emotions the phone goes again it's a message from my brother telling me he didn't want to have a meltdown in front of me and how we didn't do enough things together ending in luv u bro. That was it the switch was thrown and boom I could hold back no longer, and I just let it all out. Oh my god it was wonderful. I absolutely cried like a proper baby there were tears flowing, snot running from my nose whimpering gasps of air my hands were wet with tears and covered in snot by the time I had done it was nearly as good as an orgasm but not quite and after it subsided and I regained control all the tension, anger and sorrow I had built up had just gone. Well, there may be still some anger not so much of why me but to be honest that hadn't really been there anway, shit happens, and it's just happened to me unlucky crack on.

Until now thinking about it I haven't really felt sorry for myself. Unless you think I have after reading this, but I've been so obsessed trying to protect my family from it I think that has kept the oh woe is me away from my thought pattern. Also, I think that the fact my dad had it and I'm now fifty-six with the increase in cancer numbers it's not hard doing the maths I must have a big red flag above my head with possible cancer patient on it.

On the subject of numbers and your chances of getting the big C my mind was just pondering things and I was wondering about if prostate cancer is hereditary or not. My father has a mostly bald head and I'm following in his footsteps, but my brother has a head of hair like a thick rug. How's that work then. So, I was wondering if the prostate works the same hopefully, he will be ok, and it will miss him. That would be nice because three men in the same family getting prostate cancer would be a bit much to be fair and taking the piss, I think.

TUESDAY 12TH SEPTEMBER

I should have been at work yesterday my first day back after my four off. Due to my results, I had the day off as I would not have been able to do anything if I would have gone back to work in the afternoon. I had told my manager that it was a possibility that I wouldn't be in until Tuesday.

Tuesday morning came I had spoken to my manager last night on results day and we had formulated a plan on the best time to tell the rest of our shift mates my news. We congregate in the main workshop on the mezzanine floor in the factory. The shift that were on the previous night wait for the oncoming day shift to handover any work that may need to be completed or any information they need us to know or pass on. All my shift apart from one who was on holiday were in the workshop, so I waited for the night lads to go on their merry way before telling my shift and a few of the day-based lads who were there my news.

I just got their attention and went through my diagnosis as I had done yesterday several times already. There was a mixed reaction to be honest which is what I expected. One of the older guys probably a few years older than me was asking about symptoms and how I knew to go for the PSA test in the first place. So, I went through my story to explain how I had ended up where I am now. The interesting thing about this has been that the most asked question I have had, and it is in my opinion the most important one is, what were your symptoms and what made you go to the doctors in the first place? There were a few other people who I had worked with over the last fifteen years where I am now that I needed to tell in person which I did as quickly as I could get to them before they heard through the rumour mill. I also went and told my department boss the chief Engineer. He was a little shocked and I think he may have thought it might have been union business I wanted to talk to him about, but it obviously wasn't. He was brilliant, very supportive and told me if there was anything I needed like time off to just go see him. I have to say with being a decent size Engineering department we have had several cases of cancer while I have been working here and the company have been excellent at taking care of the Engineers needs. The current chief Engineer has been no exception and to be honest he's probably gone above and beyond while he's been in the top job. So that was probably most of the people I needed to tell, told.

I had one more person to telephone tonight before he found out from someone else. He was my golfing buddy whom I have known from being kids. I won't go into the conversation as it was similar to most of the others but not as emotional being on the phone, it was ok, but I will tell you his first comment which I thought was great considering where this all started from in the first place.

"Ohhhh knackers", he said.

WEDNESDAY 20TH SEPTEMBER 2023

Not been writing much for a few days. To be honest I have been reading through my diary and I suppose you could call it editing as there are a lot of words I've missed when I've been trying to write stuff down while it's fresh in my mind. The punctuation isn't the best either but it's a diary and it's the story not the punctuation that's important here. I've had a few messages over the last few days, and they are upsetting. I think because I haven't had to have any treatment, I don't really think it's sunk in as to how lucky I am really at this point in time.

To find out I have cancer but to find it out when it's as early as it is has been really lucky for me. Thousands of people are not that lucky.

It's not changed my life in any way yet physically but mentally my mind is racing. I think I've checked my pensions nearly every day. I am now thinking about holidays I want to go on to places I've never been before. It really is a jolt when you hear about people getting the big C but fucking hell when it's you people are hearing about that's got it, it's like being hit with a lightning bolt.

So, three things happened today at work relating to my recent joining of the big C club. Nobody had spoken to me or asked me about my diagnosis yesterday which was my first day back on shift so I was thinking most people who know me probably know by now and while I've had my days off it would have been a conversation people would have had. So far so good then like buses three come at once.

HAPPENING NUMBER ONE

This is not really something that happened I suppose but I think it's worth mentioning. More of a continuation of telling people that didn't know. I'm a union rep at work and I'm sort of the management's contact person out of the three reps we have including me. Anyway, we need another rep to replace one that packed it in. So, I'm sorting out all the paperwork and dealing with the area rep and the Engineer who's going to be the new rep. So, I go to see him, and he knows what I'm there for so we get talking about the rep's position what I'm going to do next and what will happen going forward.

"So, I don't know if you have heard anything about me on the grape vine, so I'll tell you then you hear it from the horse's mouth. I'm ok we caught it early, but I have got prostate cancer", I told him without dragging it on. I did wonder if the cancer deafness would kick in. Now I don't work with this guy on a daily basis, but we have spoken to each other plenty of times over the years since he started. He works in a different department to me, so our paths don't cross that often. Even not having that close a working relationship I could see the news shocked him. He reacted instantly on hearing "cancer". I could see in his body language and facial expression that he was upset or maybe shocked at finding out my news.

We spoke for a while and to be fair to him he was on the ball with his health and has had blood tests on several occasions on and

up to reaching his 60th year on this planet. But he wasn't sure if the bloods he had had tested were tested for PSA. We ended our conversation, and he was going to get in touch with his doctor's surgery to find out if the PSA had been checked and if not, he would be asking if he could book an appointment to have this done. Result.

HAPPENING
NUMBER TWO

It was just before dinner time and my Electrical manager came in the workshop looking a little flustered with a box in his hand.

"Stu, I think I've dropped a bollock. I'm sorry I think I've dropped you in it mate", he says.

"Oh, right why what have I done", thinking I'm getting a telling off for doing something wrong.

"So, you know when we were working on the scanners last week and you told me about you know. Well, I've told somebody I let it slip mate I never thought, and it just came out then I realise you asked me not to tell anyone", he answered very apologetically.

"Oh, right that's ok, I thought I was getting a bollocking. You had me going there for a minute I thought I was in for it", I said.

"I'm really sorry Stu", he said continuing to apologise.

"It's not a problem mate, honestly, I've told as many people now that want to listen. You can tell anybody you like it's common knowledge now. Listen if there's anyone you want to tell then tell them and tell them they can come and talk to me about it if they are worried about something. I will tell them anything they ask if I have the answer, it's not a problem mate honestly", I explained.

So, I reassured him it was general knowledge now and he could speak freely about my diagnosis, and I would willingly explain or

talk to anyone about it that was interested.
I think it will get easier for me to talk about when it is common knowledge and just another conversation especially when all the emotion of the first few weeks of finding out has calmed down.

HAPPENING
NUMBER THREE

This next happening is what makes it hard and what I mean by the initial emotion of finding out.

I had eaten my lunch and was back in the factory on my way to do some planned maintenance work. Our workshop is on a mezzanine floor and to get to the shop floor where all the machinery is, and the cakes are baked there are several sets of staircases you can use to get down there.

I had reached the bottom of one of the staircases and was just starting to walk down the side of one of the big cooling conveyors when I saw two FLLs on the other side. I won't use names again, but one was a man, and one was a woman. FLL means front line leader. I think they are called something else now after the resent re-structure but anyway. I look over and they had seen me before I saw them. The woman who I have known at work now for quite a few years is waving paperwork across her face to cool herself down and to stop what looked like could be tears forming in her eyes.

"Hi Stu, are you ok", she asked.

I looked and was not taking in what she was saying to me. She was waving papers in front of her face looking at me with big eyes that could shed tears at any moment.

"Hi, yeh I'm good how are you two", I answered.

"Ok, how are you are you alright", she asked again.

My brain then caught up and realised she wasn't asking if I was alright, she was asking if I was alright with my cancer.

"Oh, am I alright, alright you mean. You know about the, you know then", I was trying to not say the word, so she didn't get more upset.

"Yes, yes, I'm good honestly. I'm ok we've got it early I don't need treatment honestly, I'm good I really am. Thank you for asking that's much appreciated really", I called across the cooler conveyor.

She looked across, mouthed ok and waved with her free hand not wafting paper across her face as they walked away.

I have known this lady for several years not sure exactly how many, but you build up relationships with people at work and I suppose care for them in a friendship manner without realising.

I suppose it's only when something nasty happens like getting cancer or a nasty accident happens that people show how nice they are and how much friendships mean to them.

It was really touching and knocked me of my stride a bit to be honest. It's reactions like hers that really do mean a lot as they are not expected.

So, I went from the previous day not talking about the big C in any way to having three separate and different conversations about it today in one way or another.

THURSDAY 21ST SEPTEMBER 2023

I started taking the tablets I had been prescribed after my last night shift as the doctor told me to take one a night every night. I never thought to mention I work shifts. Must have slipped my mind but I can't think why, mmmm. So, I've been taking them nearly a week or so it's 8.30am and I've just been for a piss. OMG and I really mean oh my god. Have you ever had something bother you and it went on for a long time, so you just thought it was normal, but then it went away or was cured or fixed. I am really shocked and amazed at what these tablets have done. For quite a while now and I can't honestly think for how long I have had to do a little push when I need to pee. The doctor asked me about it but I've no idea for how long I've been like this. If I think hard about it, I bet it's been like that for nearly most of this year but again I'm not sure. It may have got a little worse these last few months maybe with the cancer again I'm not too sure.

So, this morning I go for a pee. I stand in position over the toilet lift the seat and I've got a bit of morning glory going on, so I make sure I take aim and I'm about to do the little push when my pee just came out. I am not kidding it was unbelievable I could not believe I didn't have to push to piss. It was awesome it just basically fell out of me like a piss waterfall. I just stood watching thinking who the fuck can make tablets that can make your double sized prostate relax so you can piss like this because you are a fuking genius.

I am not kidding, I am honestly taken aback with this. I just cannot believe how much difference these tablets have made. I just didn't want my pee to stop, it felt like the best pee I have had in my life. Today I am going to drink gallons of water just to make sure it wasn't a fluke or that I didn't dream it. I did also think about the pushing to pee being a symtom of prostate issues and it never entered my mind I could have a problem, I was just getting old.

As an Electrical Engineer I solve problems every day it's my job and I went to college to learn that job. But when I do my job, I'm using equipment that I can see in front of me. How the hell do you start designing a chemical that is going to make my prostate not squeeze my piss pipe so I can piss more freely. Absolutely amazing well done chemist tablet makers, wow.

It's well over a week now since my diagnosis and I must be honest it still hasn't sunk in the enormity of my situation and the effect it's had on my friends and loved ones. As days go by, I do find myself thinking of it less and there may be a couple of hours go by where it's not been at the front of my thoughts at all. Hopefully this length of time will get longer and longer and the mentioning of the subject less and less. The regular checks will always bring it back to the front of my thoughts, but they will be times for my wife and I to live through. People will only know about them if we choose to tell them, or they ask.

I have to say writing this diary has been something that has given me something to channel my thoughts on. I have spent many hours on this, and it has been enjoyable, scary, I wouldn't say depressing, worrying as hell, but I hope worth it.

SATURDAY 7TH OCTOBER 2023

It's been almost a month now since my diagnosis and I thought I would just put a few lines in just as a catch up on where I am now. Most of us lead a busy life with lots to do each and every day. As I have mentioned I work a four-on-four-off shift pattern. On my days off I try to do as many things as I possible can so as not to waste the time I have free by doing nothing. I have many hobbies which keep me busy. All of these are and have been a help in getting on with my life since finding out I have cancer. I have a good diagnosis which is brilliant, but I still have cancer. I have had up days and I have had down days.

I have noticed that some people have slightly changed the way they address me, but it may be in my head. After the first week or so telling everyone, it then was down to me to mentally adjust and get on without dwelling on or letting the bastard disease get me down. I have had a few bad days I would be lying if I said I haven't. I know I have been a little snappy with work mates and especially with my wife. I apologise most sincerely for this to all of you.

My wife said to me last week "don't let it control you. Your still you, live your life don't let it take over", and yes, she is right in what she says. I'm a mentally strong person and not much really bothers me. I do feel strongly about certain things, and I can get animated over these things. I don't like people who ride others, and I can and do speak my mind. I have never had cancer before and if you haven't then I am glad for you and I hope you never get it. Luckily, I have a good diagnosis, but I won't lie I have had some bad days because it is cancer.

It's not the fact that I've sat and thought about having the big C. I suppose it's more that your aware that it's there. It's in you, it's nasty, is it going to grow, is it going to kill you, is it laughing at you, it's living there rent free taking the piss causing all this pain to me, my family and friends.

My wife works different shifts including sleep overs. I have been prescribed some tablets to, as the doctor put it "improve my quality of life", but I have made the decision to stop taking them. After about two weeks on the tablets, I had noticed I was getting pains on the left side of my chest. These pains started to get worse and more regular. Two days ago, I decided to stop taking them as the pain was becoming severe and there virtually all the time. I take the tablets at nighttime and on my first day shift Thursday I was really struggling at work with the pain. I spoke to my wife Thursday evening and decided to stop taking the tablets. Yesterday after only missing one tablet the pain had gone. Totally cleared nothing, no pain at all. Was some of it psychosomatic I don't know maybe but the fact is I don't have the pain anymore. Another thing that I was feeling especially when I was in bed on my own when Terry was at work on a sleep over was anxiety. I've never been an anxious person ever, but laid in bed on my own I felt horrible. I have never felt like this before and with the chest pains it was horrendous and I hope I never feel like that again.

The mind is a powerful tool and there is a lot of information and help now available about mental health. It's been a few days now not taking the tablets and I feel ten times better, physically and mentally.

The tablets I was taking are Tamsulosin hydrochloride 400 micrograms. These were mainly to help me pass urine easier. The doctor who prescribed my medication did say to me if I feel unwell taking them, I was ok to stop taking them. They were to assist in making my life easier but the side effects I felt were making my life worse not better. My circumstances are special to me, so I do not advocate you doing as you please with your medication this is my story and my circumstances. Always consult your doctor before making any decision about altering your meds program.

I will now wait and see how not taking the tablets affects me when I go for a pee. At the moment I am still flowing unhindered, but we will see. To be honest it never bothered me having to give that little push to start my pee, but it has been nice not pushing. I know one thing; I'll take the pushing over the severe chest pains and anxiety all day.

You all know my story because I have told you it, and now my diary will come to a conclusion for now. I will continue writing but it will probably be every three months unless something else happens in between. I think I will continue to put it in this diary but mostly for myself and maybe my family. If I think, there's a diary two then maybe that may be an option I will wait and see.

CONCLUSION

This is my actual diagnosis.
Gleason 3+3 prostate cancer
Recommending staging T2A NOMO
Presenting PSA 3.5
Prostate volume 68cc with a PSA density of 0.05

Therefore, for the time being the answer to the title of this book "does it stay, or does it go" my double sized prostate gland stays where it is, inside me.

That is the official version of what I have going on in my double sized prostate gland. The doctor giving us the results mentioned my prostate is twice the size it should be, but not due to the cancer. It doesn't take long for people to forget your troubles as they have plenty of their own to worry about. There's always something in people's lives that is the next thing to talk about and that's good. I suppose it's wrong of me to say they forget because it's not a case of forgetting it's a case of not mentioning it to make me feel uncomfortable and remind me of something that I would rather not like being reminded of.

I'm not going to forget I don't think that is possible certainly not at this early stage and especially as I will be having blood tests every three month. I will carry on with my life as it isn't in anyway stopping me from doing anything which is as I've already said a great result.

If you're going to get cancer then what I have been diagnosed with is as good as it gets where prostate cancer is concerned, I suppose. There is pain virtually everday but it is minimal and bearable at this point, I don't like taking tablets and have been told by two doctors that this is a stupid attitude to have, but I can't help being who I am and doing what I do. I suppose I am old enough and wise enough now to realise that at my age medication is probably going to start creeping into my life more and more. I do believe the less you take the less you need and once you start looking at taking tablets for this pain and that ache, you're on your way out. The body is resilient, and the mind is a powerful instrument if you use it positively and not negatively. Only time will tell what happens from here and I can only hope I have lots of time left because I have lots I want to see and lots I still want to do.

Was my way of telling people my news the right way I don't know but it was my way. You will have to do it your way and there the choices you will have to make. Time has passed now nearly two weeks since finding out. If anyone asks now, I don't beat about the bush I just tell them what I have. The cancer deafness may or may not kick in, but it takes less time to explain and gets it over and done without it dragging on and becoming uncomfortable for them and for me.

GENTLEMEN IT IS SIMPLE ANY PAIN OR DISCOMFORT, IN OR NEAR YOUR KNACKERS GO TO THE DOCTORs. YOU ARE NOT BIG, STRONG OR CLEVER IF YOU DONT. IF YOU DO, IT MAY JUST SAVE YOUR LIFE.

If you have read my book, then I thank you.

If reading my book has helped you in anyway then it was worth the effort on my behalf.

I thank my wife Terry and I want her to know that I love her with all my heart she has been there for me all the way through this journey (well, from when I eventually told her, dick head that I am).

I thank all the family and friends for their support and concern they have shown me. Thank you all so much you have no idea how much that love, and concern has helped me over the last few weeks.

My Prostate gland has cancer, but it is still my Prostate gland and if I can keep it that way it will be staying exactly where it is inside me.

AFTERMATH

Your results are in it's not looking good

The big C has landed your thinking oh fuck

But glass half full it's not that bad

No chemo or radio needed so don't be sad

Your heads all mixed up you can't think straight

Just don't panic you'll lose more weight

Worry not it's the best it could be

It's not getting me fuck the big C

Up and down your emotions are raw

Sometimes I smile I think I'm all good

But sometimes I don't smile

I feel like I could cry well maybe I should

A few weeks gone by the news is still new

It will take another week maybe even a few

It will get easier when your head gets in gear

It makes it much easier now your not living in fear

You may get pissed off and snap at your mates

You may even get angry and chelp at the wife

Some might say your no different but what do they know

It's not fucking easy let me tell you so

The damage it's done
The pain it's caused
Don't let it win don't walk down its path
It's all up to you to stop the
Aftermath

Stu

Don't forget men.

GENTLEMEN IT IS SIMPLE ANY PAIN OR DISCOMFORT, IN OR NEAR YOUR KNACKERS GO TO THE DOCTORs. YOU ARE NOT BIG, STRONG OR CLEVER IF YOU DONT. IF YOU DO, IT MAY JUST SAVE YOUR LIFE

ACKNOWLEDGMENTS

I would just like to thank, my wonderful wife who puts up with every silly idea I have or project I take on, because without her this would not be the same story. My father for shoving me for the test and being my father, my parents I love you both. My Brother who was one of my early readers, along with Alan my work mate, your criticism was most welcome. James, you were there as a friend not just a good boss and came through on both counts. All friends and family for your support I thank you all most sincerely. To my doctor in the local surgery and the team at Barnsley hospital that have dealt with me from the start of this journey to where I am now. I thank you with my heart and soul you have all been amazing.

During this journey we recently lost our beloved dog Misty who had been with us for fourteen years. Misty you were a dog in a million. You were there wagging your tail to put a smile on our faces everyday. You are missed. X

ABOUT THE AUTHOR

Stuart Alexander Hayward comes from a small village in Yorkshire. He was a clever child but never really tried at school. He came into his own when he became an apprentice electrician after leaving school. At college during his apprenticeship he excelled getting top marks through most of his college years ending up with an HNC in Electrical and Electronic Engineering. He loves technology and has been a qualified Electrician for almost forty years.

Stuart met his wife Terry whilst working at the same factory. They were soon engaged, married and have two children, a girl and a boy. Both Stuart and his wife are very family orientated and love animals. At the time of writing two cats, a puppy dog and a parrot.

Stuart has many hobbies which include writing, going to the gym, riding his bicycle, playing golf, playing the guitar and playing new and old retro arcade games across many gaming platforms. He enjoys writing poems and now this his first book.

Stuart and his wife manage an allotment from the local council. This allotment has come down the generations from her Grandfather to her father and now to her. It is a decent plot of land and takes up a lot of their time.

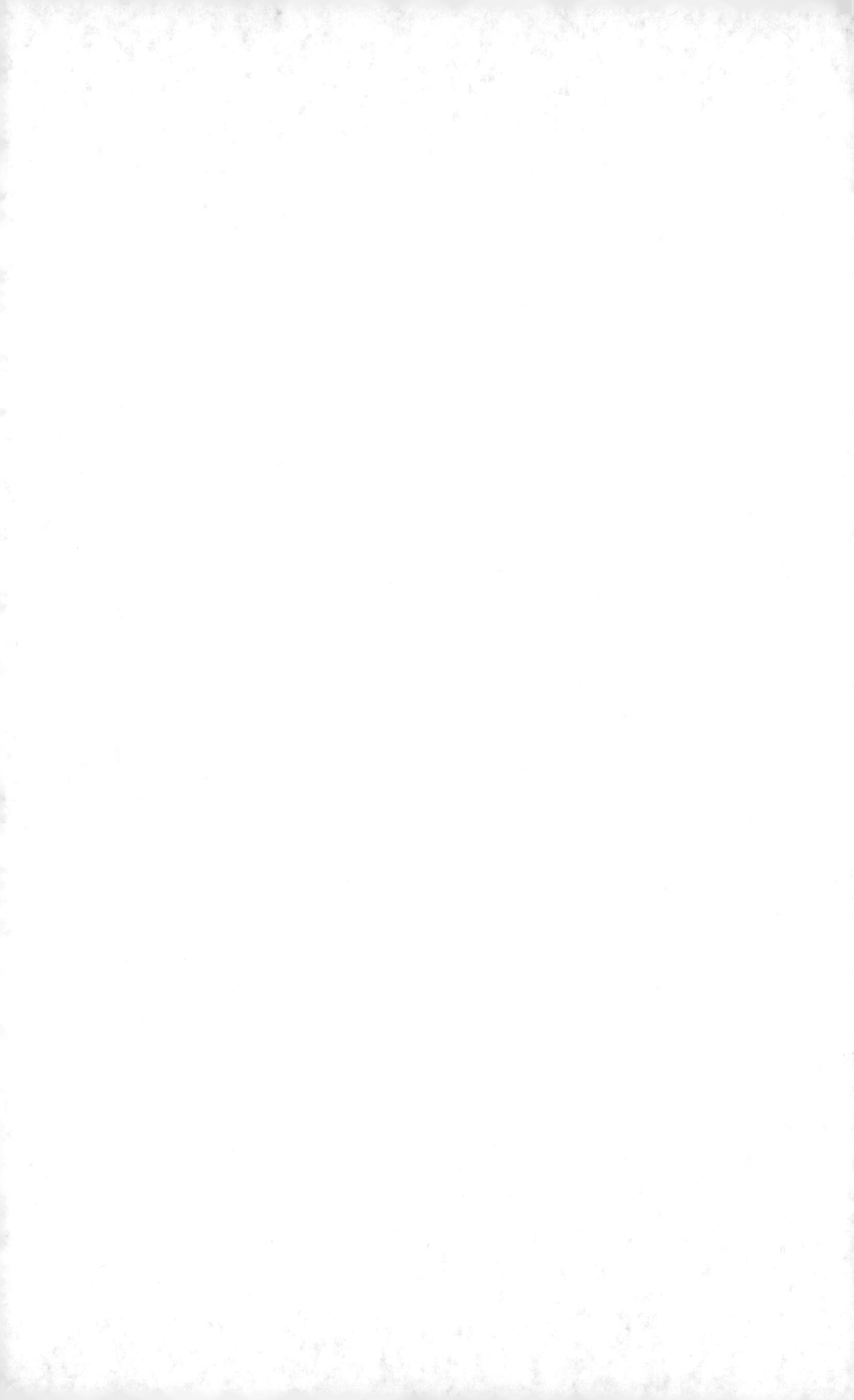

www.ingramcontent.com/pod-product-compliance
Lightning Source LLC
Chambersburg PA
CBHW070822260726
48660CB00005B/1948